Healing
Lost Souls

Also by William J. Baldwin, Ph.D.

Spirit Releasement Therapy: A Technique Manual

Past Life Therapy: A Technique Manual

CE-VI: Close Encounters of the Possession Kind

(Co-authored with the Rev. Judith A. Baldwin)

From My Heart to Yours: A Transformational
Guide to Unlocking the Power of Love

SRT Coursebook: Workbook for the
BASIC SRT Training Course

By the Rev. Judith A. Baldwin:

The Inner Knower

Healing Lost Souls

Releasing Unwanted Spirits from Your Energy Body

William J. Baldwin, Ph.D.

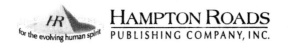

HAMPTON ROADS
PUBLISHING COMPANY, INC.
for the evolving human spirit

The term Spirit Releasement Therapy was trademarked in 1993 by the
Center for Human Relations. For convenience and clarity, the superscript
registration mark "®" will not be used in the text of this book.

Cover design by Marjoram Productions
Cover art © 2003 Ron Chapple/Thinkstock/PictureQuest

Hampton Roads Publishing Company, Inc.
1125 Stoney Ridge Road
Charlottesville, VA 22902

434-296-2772
fax: 434-296-5096
e-mail: hrpc@hrpub.com
www.hrpub.com

If you are unable to order this book from your local
bookseller, you may order directly from the publisher.
Call 1-800-766-8009, toll-free.

Library of Congress Cataloging-in-Publication Data

Baldwin, William J.
    Healing lost souls : releasing unwanted spirits from your energy body
/ William J. Baldwin.
        p. cm.
Includes bibliographical references and index.
    ISBN 1-57174-366-9 (alk. paper)
    1. Reincarnation therapy. 2. Spiritual healing and spiritualism. 3.
Spirit possession. 4. Exorcism. 5. Multiple personality--Treatment.
I. Title.
    RC489.R43B35 2003
    616.89'14--dc21

                                        2003006460

ISBN 13: 978-1-57174-366-4
10 9 8 7 6 5 4
Printed on acid-free paper in the United States

This book is lovingly and respectfully dedicated to Hazel Denning, Ph.D., Grande Dame of past-life therapy, founding president of APRT, the Association for Past-Life Research and Therapies. Moving gracefully through life with never an unkind word, you believed in me and supported my work from the beginning. Thank you, Hazel.

Contents

Preface

What exactly is consciousness? Does consciousness exist in non-physical form? What happens to me when my body dies? *Me*, the self-aware one looking out of my eyes, the "I" who remembers my whole life. Does my personality survive bodily death? What is soul? Can it be damaged? What about reincarnation? Can my soul come back again in a body of my own? Can I remember my own past lives? Can I go into another body? What is spirit possession? These are age-old questions, and no one has offered any universally acceptable answers. Nor can there be any "scientific proof" for such answers.

Most of the world's religious philosophies include some notion of life, death, survival, and rebirth, as well as some way to balance one's harmful thoughts and deeds. The Golden Rule is a perfect description of karma: "Do unto others as you would have others do unto you."

In 1970, I graduated from dental school, and until 1982, conducted my practice in southern California. In a few weekend courses, I learned hypnodontics; that is, dental hypnosis. I used my new knowledge to help my dental patients eliminate fear of the drill and the needle, to control gagging, minimize swelling, and maximize healing. Dental hypnosis works.

I continued attending other courses, both in medical hypnosis and counseling hypnotherapy. In one advanced hypnosis workshop, I personally experienced myself in a prior lifetime. It was a startling experience, and though I wasn't aware of it at the time, a life-changing event. Following that, I read what few books had been written on past-life therapy by therapists who were developing the field, and I set out to learn how to do past-life regression therapy. Past-life therapy is a safe, swift, direct approach to psychotherapy; the results are often immediate and lasting.

During a therapy session, the client is guided to locate the cause of the presenting problem, the conflict that first brought him or her into therapy. It might be childhood trauma, something that happened in the birth experience, or an event in another time and place, perhaps another lifetime. At least it often seems to be a prior life. The client will feel it as a personal experience, but in a different body. I began doing past-life therapy with clients in 1981, eighteen months before leaving the practice of dentistry.

After ten years of experience gained by conducting several thousand therapy sessions with private clients, I produced my first book, *Spirit Releasement Therapy: A Technique Manual*, a comprehensive volume on regression therapy process and technique. The rationale of regression therapy is presented in detail, with a focus on the methods of discovery, resolution, forgiveness, and healing of the unfinished business of past times that contaminate the present life experience.

A hypothetical model of the spiritual reality was developed from the narrative details of therapy sessions, at least partially consistent with historical beliefs about life after death. The techniques of past-life therapy (PLT) and spirit releasement therapy (SRT) are clearly outlined in the SRT manual. PLT and SRT are closely linked in clinical practice; a thorough knowledge of both is essential for the well-trained regression therapist.

While searching for the origin or cause of their personal problems, many clients recalled traumatic events in other lifetimes; many discovered other people as the source of conflicts and problems. Dead people. Spirits or souls of deceased humans were interfering with living people. This sounds like spirit possession.

I had much more to learn about spiritual reality and the human condition. My clients and the entities attached to them became my teachers. My comforting beliefs about the benign nature of the spirit world had to be abandoned.

Are there invisible spirits around us? Can the soul of a deceased human being interfere with a living person? Is spirit possession a real possibility in our contemporary world? Is exorcism for real? Are there really demons as described in religious literature? What is an entity?

The term "spirit possession" suggests total takeover, which sometimes happens. Entity (an individual being with real and independent existence) or spirit attachment implies connection, clinging, a parasitic invasion of the host by another conscious being. This is a more accurate description of the condition. I coined the term "spirit releasement therapy" to more realistically describe the rational, methodical, gentle process of treatment for the affliction of spirit attachment.

One section of the SRT manual is titled "Recovery of Soul-Mind Fragmentation." Inspired by the shamanic healing process of soul retrieval, recovery of soul fragmentation (RSF) is a clinical approach to the condition of soul loss. It has become an essential part of our counseling sessions for dealing with trauma in this life and any other. Again, the techniques of RSF were developed by trial and error in therapy sessions.

The SRT manual was written primarily as a textbook for professionals who wanted to use the techniques in their own healing practice with clients. The three modalities, PLT, SRT, and RSF, together constitute the Baldwin Method of regression therapy.

Some of the case histories in this new book first appeared in the SRT manual. All case descriptions are taken from records of clinical sessions with real people—normal people with common, everyday problems—with their permission, or people who volunteered for demonstration sessions in group settings. Names and some details have been changed to protect anonymity. Minor editing has been done in some dialogues for the sake of clarity.

Symptoms of physical conditions and medically diagnosed illness are often eased or eliminated through these therapies. Clients report relief from mental and emotional problems that plague so many of us: anxiety, depression, fears and uncertainties, phobias and compulsions, difficulties in relationships, unreasonable guilt and remorse, inappropriate anger and resentment, feelings of rejection and abandonment, feelings of not belonging here, and alienation from other people and society.

Soul loss as a cause of disease and the healing process of soul retrieval have been firmly lodged within the domain of shamanism. Though largely denied and ignored by traditional mental health and medical practitioners, the conditions of discarnate interference and soul fragmentation are common. A client in an altered state of consciousness can quickly and easily discover past lives, attached entities, and the voids that indicate soul loss. The treatment for these three conditions is specific and effective.

This book is not meant to be a training manual for conducting past-life therapy, spirit releasement therapy, or recovery of soul fragmentation. It was planned and written for the purpose of bringing this knowledge to everyone who is interested in the mind-body-*spirit* model of holistic healing. Past-life therapy is already a popular subject, the techniques well developed. Prior to the beginning of the twentieth century, spirit possession and exorcism were relegated to the dusty archives of medieval religious beliefs and practice. However, in the last few decades, deliverance ministry has been a growing force in the religious community. The Catholic Church has cautiously revealed more about the practice of exorcism and the growing need for the service.

Deliverance ministry continues to be a growing force in the Protestant religious community. The term "deliverance" is used in a generic sense to refer to any confrontation with an evil spirit with the purpose of overcoming its influence and "casting out" the intruder. It is taken from a phrase in The Lord's Prayer: "Lead us not into temptation, but deliver us from evil." The Bible describes Jesus and his disciples "casting out unclean spirits" during their ministry.

The clinical treatment methods for spiritual afflictions described in this book are slowly gaining public and professional acceptance. It is time for the superstition and fear surrounding reincarnation and spirit possession to be brought into the Light for healing.

In a counseling session a client describes a current problem or conflict situation. As the dialogue progresses, the client will feel sensations in the body such as tightness, tension, pain, heat, or cold. I direct the client to focus on the sensation and describe the size, shape, color, emotional tone, sound, or any words coming from the sensation.

As a person concentrates on memories, emotional feelings, and physical sensations, the consciousness alters, the subconscious mind becomes more accessible, and traumatic memories emerge. This is a self-induced mental state, a focused awareness, not produced by hypnotic suggestion. Classic hypnosis techniques are not used in this work. In this way, the client is in charge, not the therapist. As I was developing this methodology, through trial and error with much course correction, I learned a great deal by listening and learning to ask the right questions to assist in uncovering the painful, forgotten memories and the lasting impact on the person.

Once the client speaks any words from the sensation, the questions are directed to the sensation, whatever *it* is: a past-life personality of the client, an attached entity of some kind, the inner child personality, a memory of father's or mother's voice scolding them as a child, or something else. Whatever emerges is usually related to the present life problem. The memories of painful events are repressed, buried in the subconscious mind along with anger, fear, sadness, guilt, and other emotions associated with the events.

The repressed memories may be distorted, but the pain still lingers. As a therapist, I accepted what clients experienced and described as real. For them, it was real. There is no attempt at interpretation, which is an intellectual intrusion on an emotional experience. The goal of this therapy is to assist the client in uncovering the painful memory, resolving the conflicts, easing the emotional and physical pain, exercising forgiveness, and perceiving the actual nature of the original painful event. Only then is healing possible in the present time.

Cartographers in the Old World drew maps of the familiar geography of that time. In their view, the sea extended only a little way out from the European landmass. Beyond the edge of the known waters depicted on these old charts, they wrote, in careful script,

"Here there be dragons." Perhaps more truth than they could possibly know.

Explore with us some of the dimensions of consciousness we have discovered in clinical practice. You may find much of this work startling, challenging, even incredible at first. I certainly did. This book is essentially the journal of our discoveries as we have sailed this voyage through the uncharted seas of the multiverse: exploring the mystery of consciousness itself. Revelations from thousands of clients describing their spiritual reality while in altered states of consciousness have been fascinating, and have contributed to my spiritual growth and evolution. I trust this volume will have a similar effect on the reader. Read with an open mind. This is Middle America speaking. This could be any of us. It *is* some of us.

Acknowledgments

Again I acknowledge my most eloquent and profound teachers: my clients who have trusted me to explore their minds and souls, probing the raw phenomenology of human consciousness. I acknowledge the nonphysical beings who have spoken to me through the voices of their living hosts.

My curiosity continues to grow as new spiritual vistas emerge. It is a grand exploration!

I am grateful to friends who read the rough draft and offered praise and criticism, challenge and correction. Tom Saunders, long-time friend and colleague, suggested I not change a word. Our dear friend Marilyn Roofner gave of her time to read the manuscript and, with her laser-sharp perception, suggest changes and additions to clarify these subjects for newcomers to the field.

Dear friend and colleague David Ritchey, true to his ruthless quest for accuracy, challenged concept, context, and content. John Williams, another respected friend, volunteered to read and edit the manuscript, resulting in significant changes to the work.

Richard Leviton, senior editor at Hampton Roads Publishing Company, applied the final polish to the book. I was delighted with his comment on the first draft: "Excellent book. Well done." My intention is that this book make a difference in the world.

And to you, my beloved Judith, partner in life, in our love, and in the work, I again pledge my eternal love. I am grateful for every moment we have shared and will share together, here and beyond. My life and my soul are richer for our joining. Namasté.

Introduction

Classic hypnosis is usually understood as a sleeplike trance usually induced by a hypnotist. In the hypnotic state, a person may experience forgotten or suppressed memories, hallucinations, and heightened suggestibility. A hypnotic state can also be brought on by boredom, as in a long, uneventful automobile ride, or by daydreaming in a boring classroom.

A hypnotherapist—that is, a psychotherapist who uses hypnosis—can induce this mental state and proceed to ease chronic pain, eliminate fear of treatment such as dental procedures, or uncover suppressed traumatic memories that affect a client's life. Age regression is a technique of hypnotherapy used to uncover and treat childhood trauma. Sexual dysfunction often stems from repressed early memories.

The study of hypnosis, hypnotherapy, and the use of altered states of consciousness[1] naturally led to the discovery of past-life regression. As a client is guided to recall the source of a problem or conflict, the memory retrieved might be in this life or an earlier incarnation. The alert therapist can recognize the difference and proceed with appropriate treatment.

The first book on past-life recall through hypnosis was written by a Frenchman, Col. Albert de Rochas, in 1911.[2] The first American work was self-published in 1942 by Asa Martin and focused on the spiritual aspects of the experience.[3] Ron Hubbard's methods of Dianetics uncovered past-life traumatic memories.[4]

In 1956, Morey Bernstein's book, *The Search for Bridey Murphy*, was published. It was the account of a Colorado housewife who recalled, under hypnosis, what seemed to be a past life in a small village in Ireland. Details of the village life were later confirmed by careful investigation, though debunkers rejected this information and tried to refute the findings of the investigators. Bernstein's book and the subsequent movie were very successful. Through popular media, the notion of the cycle of rebirth was introduced to the American public. Several books on past-life therapy were published in the late 1970s.[5]

Reincarnation is an integral part of Eastern spiritual beliefs, yet the concept has been eliminated in Western religious thinking. Four fifths of the religious teachings of the world include the concept of reincarnation and karma. It is presented as part of the spiritual path of human beings. Reincarnation and karma offer a path of balancing past misdeeds through personal responsibility. When the notion of reincarnation was voted out of Christian teachings, the church fathers usurped personal responsibility of the people and became the authority over human salvation, redemption, and any possibility of spiritual evolution.

The possibility of survival of consciousness following physical death is a primary focus of some investigators in this field. No matter how many people describe the experience, such reports are considered anecdotal, therefore not worthy of scientific scrutiny. There is no *scientific* proof that the personality or human consciousness survives death of the body, yet more than 11 million people have gone through the near-death experience, or NDE, and reveal similar descriptions.[6]

Personal experience of past-life recall is beyond the scope of scientific research. Although some investigators have documented facts and information retrieved in past-life recall, this does not prove reincarnation. However, past-life therapy, based on these concepts, is effective in relieving many human conditions, mental and physical. Therapists and counselors in many parts of the world ease the suffering of their clients with these techniques. Memories of traumatic events from former lives seem to affect the present life. Burning at the stake or being stoned to death by a crowd can induce a fear of public speaking, the most common phobia. Drowning in a prior lifetime can cause a fear of water. A crushed skull *then* can produce chronic headaches *now*. Damaged internal organs caused by accident or being mauled by a wild animal can lead to conditions like diabetes, which is caused by a poorly functioning pancreas. Details of such cases are included in the book to illustrate the techniques of past-life therapy.

A person with dissociative identity disorder (DID), formerly called multiple personality disorder (MPD), appears to have several different and distinct personalities that emerge separately and take control of the body.[7] Some of the alter personalities claim to be past-life personalities of the person; some claim to be separate entities and not part of the person at all. A few claim to be spirit guides or helpers.

The personality of a human being is the face or the mask of soul consciousness during one's lifetime. Past-life personalities tend to be dormant within the unconscious mind of a living person. In an altered state of consciousness, what some people call a hypnotic state, most people can recall previous experiences of living on Earth: sometimes in a male form; sometimes in a female form.

As a client narrates a past-life death, the past-life personality seems to remain intact. It maintains its own behaviors and addictions, physical signs and symptoms of disease, emotional distress and upsets, and attitudes. These conditions may well be carried into future incarnations for possible resolution and healing.

If this disembodied personality, the soul of a newly deceased person, fails to reach the Light, or Heaven, and instead follows or attaches to a living person, it can inflict such behaviors, symptoms, and conditions on the host. As we learn more about past-life influence, soul fragmentation, and discarnate interference, the obvious and unsettling question becomes: "Who am I?"

This question becomes vitally important as we witness an expanding model of human consciousness. Past-life trauma can lead to chronic, even fatal, illness in the present. Relationships may be affected by past-life personal interactions. Soul fragmentation and loss can contribute to depression, attention deficit, poor memory, and fatigue. Discarnate human entities can interfere with any aspect of human life. Attitudes and beliefs, phobias and emotional upset, behavior, addictions, and relationship problems are just a few areas that can be influenced. Sudden change of behavior following an accident, illness, surgery, organ transplant, even death of a family member, can indicate a new entity attachment. Dark force entities can generate anger, rage, violence, and criminal behavior.

Trance channeling or mediumship, the control of a living person by the spirit of a nonphysical teacher or a deceased human bringing a message to surviving loved ones, is an example of *voluntary* possession. The channel or medium *allows* another being to take control of the mind, voice, and body for a specified purpose and limited duration.[8] The problem is, an opportunistic discarnate entity may not want to leave at the end of the channeling session.

The condition of spirit possession, the *involuntary* takeover of a living human being by a discarnate spirit, has been described throughout recorded history. It is an affliction that can be confusing and disruptive. It can lead to death. In clinical practice with many clients, I began to understand this condition as spirit interference or *spirit attachment* rather than *spirit* or *demon possession.*

Historically, the treatment for spirit possession consisted of extracting or casting out the intruding spirits, using rituals and incantations. This duty has been assigned to the shaman, holy man, healer, or priest of both indigenous and civilized populations.

The early Chinese, Egyptians, Hebrews, and Greeks believed mental disorders were caused by demons that had taken possession of unfortunate individuals. In the New Testament, many of the healings attributed to Jesus described casting out unclean spirits.

Cases of possession are well documented throughout history. However, they are considered anecdotal, that is, without scientific verification. Experience, no matter how many humans have the same experience, does not establish scientific proof.

William James, considered by many to be the father of American psychology, seemed to accept the possibility of discarnate interference.

The refusal of modern "enlightenment" to treat "possession" as a hypothesis to be spoken of as even possible, in spite of the massive human tradition based on concrete experience in its favor, has always seemed to me a curious example of the power of fashion in things scientific. That the demon-theory will have its innings again is to my mind absolutely certain. One has to be "scientific" indeed to be blind and ignorant enough to suspect no such possibility.[9]

Thus, the scientific method will never be sufficient to explore thoroughly the depth of human consciousness. Research must include the spiritual dimension. Human experience is subjective and cannot be weighed, measured, or duplicated on demand. Yet human experience is appropriate and essential data for a comprehensive understanding of consciousness, despite the matter of "scientific proof."

William James urged that science should be based *only* on experience, and that *nothing* within the totality of human experience should be excluded from being a potential topic of scientific investigation. In his *Essays in Radical Empiricism*, James defined this term:

To be radical, an empiricism must neither admit into its construction any element that is not directly experienced, nor exclude from them any element that *is* directly experienced.[10]

At this point in the investigation of consciousness, the question of survival of the human personality after physical death remains unanswered.[11] There are many indications of survival, yet there are no tools for adequate exploration. The focus of this inquiry must be: What survives? And the ultimate question remains: What is consciousness? Is conscious awareness merely the result of biochemical processes in the brain? Or is it the essence of creation?

This exploration makes for fascinating speculation, yet the answers are elusive. The present avenues of scientific inquiry will fall short. The solution to these speculations does not lie within the three-dimensional time-space continuum.

In regression therapy, the client is guided to recall from subconscious memory the origin, the source, the cause of present life problems. This typically involves memories of traumatic events prior to the present moment, most often found in other lifetimes.

Physical and emotional trauma can apparently cause loss of soul fragments. Such trauma and the lost soul fragment can be discovered in this or an earlier lifetime. Past-life therapy can assist in healing this condition.

The techniques used to locate the source of a current problem can also lead to the discovery of an attached entity that is causing the problem. This, also, can involve the present or former lifetimes. The entity or entities are carefully and permanently released to the Light.

The clinical model of regression therapy including past-life recall, spirit releasement, and recovery of soul fragments must remain a working hypothesis without scientific proof. Even without such proof, the methods can be learned and used by other counselors with equally successful results.

This methodology cannot prove the concepts of reincarnation and karma, the existence of the human soul, the survival of personality following death, or the condition of possession of living people by discarnate entities. Yet therapy sessions often bring immediate and permanent relief from symptoms and conditions that have plagued people for years. This is the value of the work.

Nor can the techniques and methods described be considered a substitute for appropriate medical or psychological treatment in cases of actual physical or mental/emotional damage. Past-life therapy, spirit releasement therapy, and recovery of soul fragmentation cannot be considered a panacea for all the ills of humanity. However, these are the correct tools if a present life problem results from unresolved emotional issues carried over from a previous lifetime, an attached entity of some kind, or the condition of soul fragmentation.

In 1989, I met and married Judith. Rev. Judith A. Baldwin joined me in my life and work. Judith is blessed with the spiritual gifts of discernment: clairvoyance, clairaudience, and clairsentience.[12] She uses these abilities in counseling sessions with clients, confirming much of what I learned in eight years of working with clients plagued by discarnate interference. She can perceive discarnate entities of all kinds, determine the degree of soul fragmentation, and gather information regarding past-life carryover of unfinished business.

This has been a welcome contribution for me as well as a powerful healing agent for clients in our practice. She is a skilled counselor. In the individual sessions I did before working with Judith, I use the pronoun "I," in the ones following, the pronoun "we" is used.

As a therapist, I am sensitive to the client's feelings, memories, and experience, no matter how far from consensus reality the stories range. I have seen and listened to human pain; it is real. The exploration of human consciousness may uncover anything. Yet much of what is uncovered would be rejected by science. A large part of human experience lies outside the parameters of the scientific method.

Particularly in Western civilization, science and spirit finally parted company between the middle of the nineteenth century and the beginning of the twentieth century. Metaphysical and spiritual phenomena, subjects of belief and faith and therefore unprovable, were relegated to the province of religion, a great loss to the helping professions and to the human race.

Yet people continue to have mystical and spiritual experiences. Can this all be imagination or mass delusion? Déjà vu, past-life memories, out-of-body experience, near-death experience, possession by other beings or entities, channeling, psychic abilities, precognitive knowledge, UFO contact and abduction, and many other nonscientific events continue to be reported by intelligent, credible people.[13]

In our counseling practice, most of our clients through the years have discovered discarnate interference. Many firmly stated they had never before believed in such a thing, yet the direct experience is hard to deny. I could not pass it off as imaginary, the result of paranoia or delusional thinking. As a scientifically oriented investigator, I recognized and observed this phenomenon, and formed a hypothesis that was not unlike historical descriptions of spirit possession.[14] Certainly I was not the first to discover this condition in living humans.

Through clinical experience I discovered what appeared to be three main types of intrusive entity: (1) the Earthbound soul (EB), which includes deceased humans, terminated pregnancies, and mind fragments of living people; (2) the dark force entity (DFE), which includes the classic demon; and (3) the extraterrestrial (ET), which includes aliens and otherworldly beings. This book focuses primarily on these three types, though there are many other interfering entities and energies.

Spirit possession or control by a nonphysical entity goes against our most basic human and spiritual rights. It is a possibility both terrifying and preposterous. We rail against excessive political or police power. We have laws against intruders who violate our physical person or property. Medical science has developed remedies for many of the microorganisms that invade our bodies and cause disease.

We can and must expand our awareness of the nonphysical intruders. Perhaps they are the most insidious because they are invisible, overlooked, and ignored by most people. Effective methods for dealing with many of these unseen forces have been developed through trial and error.

You will find in these pages real cases of men, women, and children who have suffered with discarnate interference, often for many years. In session they discover the cause or origin of current problems, whether it is childhood trauma, past-life events, or entity attachment. Soul fragmentation and loss following a painful experience can seriously impair one's ability to live life fully. You can follow the treatment for these conditions, and see the often surprising results.

Don't be surprised if some of the cases and client reports hit close to home. These chapters cover a wide range of problems and situations that many people have encountered in this human experience. The material presented here suggests a greater, nonphysical reality, a spiritual reality. This may validate an ancient mystical teaching: each of us is a conscious being, an eternal point of consciousness, a spark of Light extended from Creator Source, and for this little time journeying in a physical body.

– 1 –

Spirit Attachment

Dan clutched his chest and left arm with his right hand. His flushed face contorted with pain, tears squeezed from his eyes. He appeared to be suffering a heart attack right there in front of me. I was stunned. At that point I had to make a choice between calling 911 or trusting the process. I trusted the process.

Robust and healthy, Dan was thirty-eight years old, yet had suffered with symptoms of heart trouble, including chest pains, for some years. Thinking it might be a past-life trauma, he wanted to explore this condition through regression therapy. As he probed his subconscious for the cause, I thought we might have uncovered a traumatic memory of another time and place. Or, he might be having a real heart attack. I shuddered at the thought.

In a few moments, Dan slumped in the recliner chair, his face relaxed and smooth. His right hand dropped to his lap. I checked his lips to see if they were turning blue. I watched his breathing. Lips remained pink, chest continued to rise and fall with each rhythmic breath. He was okay; I was greatly relieved. We continued.

Dr. Baldwin: "What just happened?"

Client: "I just died."

Dan spoke in a calm voice, with only a hint of surprise.

Next, I asked my favorite therapy question:

Dr. B.: "What happens next?"

Something always happens next. It's a safe bet. A safe question in a therapy session.

The one who had the heart attack was an older man who had lived in Hawaii. He died suddenly on the beach during his evening stroll, just as suddenly as Dan's brief "heart attack" episode only moments ago. A past life? Death in a prior lifetime? Possibly. It would not be unusual for such a past-life death to affect him in present time.

We continued.

Dr. B.: "What happens next?"

After leaving his body, the fellow hung out on the beach, unaware of time passing, unaware he had died. He was confused. This is typical behavior for an Earthbound (EB) soul of a newly deceased human. I suspected this EB had attached to Dan. The words and descriptions of what happened are the words and memory of the EB, coming through Dan's voice. An entity influences the thinking of the client, who usually does not know the difference. The details of the narrative confirm the presence of an attached spirit, an entity.

The man, as a spirit, saw a little kid getting on a school bus near the beach. The little kid was Dan at six years of age. This could have been a day after the man's death, or a year, or ten, or fifty years. That information was not essential in this session.

For some reason the older man was drawn to the child and joined Dan, apparently in the area of his heart. We could have explored the connection between them, possibly from another lifetime they shared in some way. But for the moment it was more appropriate to release Dan from the emotional and physical residue caused by this parasitic spirit attachment.

The EB was fixated in his own death throes, reliving the painful experience over and over again, repeatedly imposing on Dan the painful heart attack symptoms that were part of his body memory of dying. It had nothing to do with Dan. Medical examinations had never revealed any organic cause for the symptoms that had plagued Dan. It was more than psychosomatic; it was psycho-spirituo-somatic.

The psyche of the attached spirit was imposing the painful physical sensations on Dan's body.

With clarification of his situation, the spirit of the old man agreed to go. He was released into the Light. Most Earthbound souls don't consciously want to harm the host; they are often confused and don't know what's happening.

Dan was scheduled the next day with his doctor for a reassessment of his condition. The nurse who took his blood pressure and checked his lung volume kidded him about earning a gold star. His tests were normal for the first time since his initial appointment with the cardiologist. There were no more signs or symptoms of heart trouble, no more chest pain for Dan.

In 1980 I attended a lecture on past-life therapy by Dr. Edith Fiore. During her presentation, Dr. Fiore mentioned the problems caused by spirits of deceased human beings interfering with living people. I was incredulous. She was serious. Spirit possession was real, and she treated the condition. Wait a minute! This is the stuff of horror movies like *The Exorcist*. As she revealed in her lecture, it was also part of her psychotherapy practice.

Dr. Fiore recommended a book by Annabel Chaplin entitled *The Bright Light of Death,* which described this condition from the viewpoint of a psychotherapist. Chaplin described a number of cases of discarnate entities interfering with people. Her approach consisted of releasing these entities from the living people and sending them on to a bright light. The results with her clients seemed miraculous.

I was deeply affected by this book. The first few chapters had a powerful impact on my understanding of reality. I had to set the book aside. Though the idea that spirits could be the cause of mental and physical illness in living people was new and foreign to me, I somehow knew it was true. My personal reality was forever shifted.

More than a month passed before I was able to pick up the book again and finish reading it. The effect on me was profound, and I knew the course of my life and the nature of my life's work had taken a new direction. My natural curiosity led me to other books on the subject of spirit possession and exorcism, or "spirit releasement," as I eventually termed the work.[1] A year later, I began seeing clients for past-life therapy. With eyes to see and ears to hear, I soon discovered and recognized the signs and symptoms of attached entities.

While there were a number of books on past-life therapy available by that time, there were none that described and outlined a rational, methodical clinical approach to relieving the condition of spirit possession. As a scientifically trained and educated health professional, I needed such a methodology. Eventually I discovered that treatment of the human mind and soul provided a clinical approach in a spiritual context.

Religious texts accepted a preconceived notion of demons. The classic adversarial approaches to exorcism were steeped in ritual and superstition. The accepted method of exorcism seemed violent and without compassion. I could not accept this. As a result, I rejected the traditional religious approaches of both exorcism and deliverance ministry and sought a more gentle approach.

Dr. Carl Wickland, a psychiatrist and an avid Spiritualist, published his first book, *Thirty Years Among the Dead*, in 1924. The volume described his work, which he called "depossession." The spirits who afflicted his patients were invited to channel through his wife, Anna, a gifted medium. His conversational approach was practical, methodical, and compassionate. He gently guided each spirit to the awareness of its own death, then invisible helpers from the spirit world assisted the confused Earthbound soul to find its rightful place in the Light. It was not necessary for the patient to be present in the treatment room. I studied his work and used it with my clients. I coined a new term for this process of mediumistic work: "remote spirit releasement."

Wickland's methods were the basis for techniques I developed in my own practice. In most cases I work directly with the client, the one with the problem of spirit attachment. I can conduct the remote spirit release through the client as the medium or connecting link to the target person, a family member or loved one. Remote spirit releasement is very successful in removing attached entities from people at a distance, much as it was in Wickland's time.[2]

Several books have been published on the use of pendulums for psychically discovering and releasing attached entities. However, since I have only rudimentary psychic ability, I chose to explore and develop a clinical approach I could understand, use effectively, and teach others to use.[3]

What happens to those newly deceased souls who try but cannot return to their own body? Can souls really get lost, unable to find the Light? Can a disembodied personality "haunt" houses and other places? Can they hang around and bother living people? Can discarnate entities affect relationships between people? Can spirit possession be real?

The answer is a resounding—and disturbing—yes. Lost souls are found in haunted houses, cemeteries, battlefields, and sites where natural disasters have occurred such as earthquakes, floods, and volcanoes. And many Earthbound souls are attached to normal, living individuals like you and me.

Our language contains numerous references to spirit interference. Think of the many statements people make:

"Something just came over me."

"I don't know what got into me."

"I am beside myself with anger!"

"I am not myself today."

"It was like I was watching myself do that. It just wasn't me!"

"When I looked into the mirror, I saw someone else's face!"

"What possessed you to do that?"

The condition of spirit possession—that is, full or partial takeover of a living human by a discarnate being—has been recognized or theorized in every age and every culture. In 90 percent of societies worldwide there are records of possession-like phenomena.[4]

Clinical evidence suggests that discarnate entities can and do influence living people. This condition has been called "possession," "possession state," "spirit possession syndrome," "spirit obsession," and "spirit attachment."[5] More recently, the term "dissociative trance disorder" was included in an appendix of the *DSM-IV*, the *Diagnostic and Statistical Manual of the American Psychiatric Association*, fourth edition. The APA establishes the diagnostic criteria and terminology for mental disorders in this country. The definition of the disorder is a clear description of entity possession.[6]

People have discovered and described many different types of nonphysical entities and energies such as: crystals; shapeless black blobs; thought forms; various types of human and nonhuman spirits; "little people" such as trolls, imps, gnomes, devas, which are the nature spirits associated with plants (this is often found with cocaine or marijuana addiction); damaged souls of victims of genetic experimentation; implants of various kinds; and other unidentifiable objects and energies.

Many people have the mistaken belief that there must be some bizarre outward signs caused by an interfering spirit as depicted in scenes from *The Exorcist*. Incidentally, the movie was based on a true case, but some of the symptoms and behaviors portrayed actually came from two other cases, combined for dramatic impact. The incidence of such violent demonic possession as is displayed in that movie is rare.[7]

In clinical practice, the aware counselor will frequently discover a condition that can best be described as spirit or entity attachment. The term possession implies total takeover of the victim/host; entity attachment causes interference with normal function and can influence behavior.

The condition is very common, and it seems that almost any trauma can cause a vulnerability to entity attachment. Some investigators in this field estimate that between 50 percent and 100 percent of the population are affected or influenced by one or more discarnate spirit entities at some time during their lives.[8] Yet most people manage to live reasonably successful lives, even in the face of such interference. Through the years, I continue to be inspired by the indomitable human spirit.

While there are many different kinds of nonphysical beings and energies that can interfere with the living, the most common are the human soul and the nonhuman entity. Human souls include the spirit of the terminated pregnancy and the mind fragment of a living person. Nonhuman entities include the classic demon, described in religious literature, and the extraterrestrial, or otherworldly being.

Human Entities

The Earthbound Human Soul

The Earthbound soul, usually described as an Earthbound (EB), the surviving consciousness of a deceased human, seems to be the most common type of discarnate entity attached to living people. Attached souls of different age groups behave differently. An old and feeble person may act confused and lost, and just as feeble in spirit as they were in real life. Some women may present themselves as maternal and nurturing, sexy, angry, secretive, or helpless and whining as they were when living. Some young men may be arrogant, hostile, domineering, challenging, controlling, as macho as if they still had their own strong male bodies.

Like any teenager, the newly deceased spirit of an adolescent is caught between childhood and adulthood when the child personality is disintegrating and the adult personality is forming. Usually a person at this age has little orientation toward the spiritual side of existence, and is often defiant toward authority figures, yet aware and even resentful that they need their elders to survive. This is a difficult time in life and even more difficult in death. The newly deceased spirit wants to stay near the grieving parents, yet wants to be free. However, they usually don't know where to go.

Earthbound souls of children often appear frightened and confused about what happened to them, where they are, lonely without mother, and cautious about talking to a stranger including the therapist. They can't understand why their parents don't come. They hide and often hesitate to speak.

These entities can become enmeshed in the aura, the energy field around the body. According to yoga philosophy, there are seven major chakras, or centers of consciousness, in the body, which lie along the spine and are associated with various physical, mental, and emotional aspects of human behavior. The base chakra, associated with the color red, lies at the base of the spine and has to do with survival and baser instincts. The second is the center of sexual and generative energy; the color is orange. The solar plexus is the seat of power, control, will, with yellow color. The heart is the center of unconditional love and is associated with green, the healing color. The throat chakra is concerned with creativity and expression and has the color blue. The brow chakra, associated with the pituitary, is called the Ajna center, or third eye, and has to do with inner seeing, intuition, and has the color indigo. The crown chakra is at the top of the head, associated with the pineal gland, and is considered the location of connection with the God-consciousness, with the color violet.

The emotional or physical trauma endured by a person can render those energy centers vulnerable. They are opened like doors to allow entry and attachment by an entity. This can be discovered in past lives or in the present. An entity can attach to any chakra, or energy center of the body.[9]

They can also attach to the surface of the body, to any interior space, or to any organ, as in cases of heart or other organ transplant.[10] The soul of the organ donor can follow the transplanted organ into the new body. Multiple organ donations from a deceased person to several people can cause a fragmentation of the newly deceased soul, as a soul fragment follows each organ to its new destination. Grateful organ recipients may get more than anticipated.

Organ Transplant

Sharon wanted to attempt a remote spirit releasement for Don, her husband, who had just undergone a heart transplant. Denise, their teenage daughter, had stayed with him in the recovery room following surgery. As he regained consciousness his first words to her were angry and scolding. It was unlike him to treat her in this manner, and her feelings were hurt. He did not seem like himself.

In the session, I directed Sharon to visualize Don. Immediately she felt a physical sensation of tightness in the chest. She repeated the first words that came into her mind:

C. (Client): "It's too tight in here. It's too tight, I can't breathe."

Questions revealed that these words belonged to Alex, the young man who was the heart donor. Alex and some friends were playing Russian roulette. Alex lost; he shot himself in the head and he died instantly. His mother was grief-stricken; his father was angry at the stupidity of the act. They accompanied the body to the hospital. They gave permission to use the organs for transplantation.

Alex was baffled by the episode. It had happened so fast, he did not yet understand. He watched the surgeons removing his organs. Alex's words came through Sharon's voice.

C.: "My kidneys went one way, my liver went another way, and my heart went somewhere else. I followed my heart because that's where I live."

His first awareness of the destination of his heart came when he saw Don on the operating table with his chest cut open and his heart missing. Alex was physically larger than Don so there was less space in the chest cavity. This was the cause of the sensation of tightness first expressed in the session.

In his fear and confusion, Alex had spoken harshly to Denise when he first saw her at her father's bedside in the recovery room. Naturally, Denise assumed her father was angry with her. It was actually Alex.

Alex was eager to leave when he understood the situation. I asked him if there were any other spirits present. An entity can often be helpful in this way. He said he could see the scars where other EBs had been attached but they left when the man "died." The entities had interpreted the removal of the heart as the death of the body.

While the original, rightful soul is out of the body during the period of clinical death, another entity can move in, invited or not. During this time attached entities might exit like rats leaving a sinking ship.

There was a change in Don following the remote releasement. He apologized to Denise for his behavior, though he did not understand why he had been angry. He assumed it had something to do with the anesthetic and other drugs. Sharon did not inform him of the remote work.

An entity can affect the limbs or hands, causing shaking, weakness or strength. In those extremely rare cases of inspirational possession[11] a discarnate being can impart knowledge, literary skills, musical ability, and artistic ability.

What would cause a newly deceased spirit to stay here near the physical world instead of going into the Light, the Heavenly place, that is so beautiful and inviting? The EB can be bound to the Earth plane by the emotions and feelings connected with a sudden traumatic death.

Clarence and the Ghost

John, an electrical engineer, discovered an attached entity named Clarence. Clarence had died as he crashed the automobile he was driving. He described getting out of the car, only to see his body still inside. Confused, he glanced around. The first thing he saw was his Aunt Agnes. This frightened Clarence, because he knew she was dead and he thought he was seeing a ghost. He had no way of knowing she was coming to guide him to the Light. He took off in the opposite direction, running into John and getting stuck. In conversation, we helped ease his fear and carefully guided him back to Aunt Agnes, who took him home to the Light.

The Baptist Minister

Many EBs discovered with my clients are controlled by their fervent religious beliefs. Some fear they will not be welcome in Heaven because of their "sins."

One male client discovered his father, who had attached after his death more than ten years earlier. His father was a devout Baptist minister with firm beliefs about the nature of Heaven. Yes, he shouted through the voice of the client, of course he had seen the Light when he died, but he wasn't about to go to Heaven until it was the way he knew it was supposed to be. In talking through this with him, he finally relented and allowed himself to be escorted lovingly into the Light.

The Soldier's Impossible Promise

Some people seem to be alone in life and cannot maintain a relationship. Some are desperate to be in a relationship with a significant other; many have no need and are not interested. It seems as if they don't feel alone or lonely or don't care about outside companionship. However, a jealous husband can remain with his wife following his death to ward off other potential lovers, as this case shows.

Louella attended a lecture I gave on the subject of regression therapy and spirit releasement. She then scheduled an appointment to check it out for herself; she had a feeling she might be affected by an attached entity.

During the initial interview, thirty-five-year-old Louella described her lonely life. She could not seem to maintain a relationship with a man for more than three months. For a client who wants to explore specifically for an attached entity, I often use the Sealing Light Meditation[12] as an invocation of light and induction into the altered state. Then I ask directly if there is someone else present. In this case we didn't even have to ask.

As Louella settled back in the recliner, she offered one more piece of information.

Client: "Oh, by the way, I had polio when I was two. Sometimes my right leg bothers me and I have muscle spasms."

In a session, the offhand remark, the "Oh, by the way . . ." statement is often the key to the core issue.

Dr. B.: "All right, focus deep inside. Locate that spark of Light at your very center."

C.: "*Ooh!* My head. It hurts!"

She grimaced and grabbed her head with both hands. She sat upright in the recliner. I recognized this as a manifestation of an attached entity, trying to get our attention. It worked.

Dr. B.: "Come out of her head! Stop hurting her! Come out of her head! We know you are here. Stop hurting her!"

The pain stopped, and Louella took her hands from her head. She lay back in the recliner. A moment later, her right leg lifted off the chair, her foot about eighteen inches above the ottoman.

C.: "This is what happens when I'm in bed with a boyfriend. My leg spasms. It always happens after we make love. It's that polio!"

The physical sensation had shifted from pain in the head to muscle spasm in the leg. A sensation that moves around in the body indicates the presence of an entity. It was her husband from a lifetime in Egypt, around A.D. 550. He had gone to war across the Mediterranean, promising to return to her. This is the soldier's impossible promise.

Her husband kept his promise, but only after he was killed in battle. He had found her in successive incarnations and had attached forty-two times. He felt justified in this, keeping his promise made to his beloved. This was definitely a distortion of love.

Millions of men have died in battles through the ages, leaving wives and sweethearts alone and desolate. Many of their souls have returned and attached to their loved ones, finding them in lifetime after lifetime. Finally, when they realize the damage they have inflicted by fulfilling their promise, they reluctantly agree to leave.

C.: "She's my wife. She's mine. I don't want her to be with any other men."

These were his words through her voice. He was trying to kick the other men out of her bed by causing spasms in the leg. After they spoke together, each through Louella's voice, and expressed the love they had felt in that Egyptian lifetime, he was finally willing to leave. His presence was not appropriate. He loved her enough to leave.

Louella returned several weeks later for another session. She wasn't aware of anything that had changed as the result of releasing the Earthbound soul of her former husband. However, several of her close friends had called to schedule private sessions. They had seen a great change in her. Whatever it was that caused the change, they wanted some of that for themselves.

Children are not immune to entity attachment. Many people who die in hospitals will actually "check out" newborns like new models in an auto dealer's showroom. Confused about their death and reincarnation, the newly deceased soul can attach to an infant. Many clients have discovered such EBs in counseling session. They are not malicious, just confused.

The reverse can happen as well. Souls of infants and children can attach to other children or adults. A young child EB discovered by an adult female client, described the moment of attaching. The client was about six years old and she was playing jacks alone, enjoying herself. She glowed with happiness. The EB had died traumatically and longed for such happiness. She just "came in" to the little girl happily playing jacks.

In session, a sixty-two-year-old male client discovered an attached female entity who died in the hospital of a lower abdominal infection. She joined him at age six following an appendectomy. The similarity of the lower abdominal infection was like a magnet to the newly deceased soul. The story within the man's family was that he never smiled following his surgery. The woman's negative characteristics affected the man's personality from the age of six.

A mother who dies when her children are young can feel such guilt that she will remain attached to each of them in a misguided attempted to stay and help them mature. An elderly mother can actually fragment before death, and a part of her will attach to each child following her death. Even a young mother who feels inadequate to her task of motherhood, anxious to "do it right," may fragment a part of herself to be with her new baby. It is a sort of unconscious baby monitoring system.

A Family Situation

A demonstration session conducted with a young woman during a class revealed an interesting twist. Gwen, the subject, was well aware of the presence of Richie, her brother, who had died in an automobile accident some months earlier. The single car accident is often a suicide.[13] She loved him deeply and welcomed him to join her after his death. He was guided to scan past lives and discovered they had been lovers in other times.

With little explanation of his situation and the effect he had on his sister, Richie was ready to separate from her and move into the Light. However, it appeared to be too far away. This indicates there is unfinished business with the host, soul fragmentation, or a nested entity, an entity within an entity. This happens when a person with an attached entity dies. The first attached entity remains within. If that newly deceased soul attaches to someone else, it still has the first attached entity "nested" within itself. If that someone else dies with the nested entities, and attaches to still another person, there is a three-layered nesting of entities.

There was no resistance on the part of either of them to the release, which indicated interference by another attached entity. As Richie explored within, he discovered the entity with him, but could not identify it.

In such cases, the focus of the questions shifts to this nested entity who responds to questioning, and Gwen gave voice to the entity. Frequently the client won't release control of their own voice and will precede the words of the attached entity with "He/she says . . ." This works just as well as actually channeling the words of the entity.

My voice was firm and demanding as I asked the following:

Dr. B.: "You, the one inside Richie, inside Gwen, step forward and speak. You, the one interfering with these people, speak up."

C.: "Yes, what do you want?"

Dr. B.: "Who are you and what are you doing here?"

C.: "I'm their mother."

I was taken aback by this revelation and immediately softened my voice for the next questions. You shouldn't speak so boldly to someone's mother.

She then revealed that she had attached when Richie was about two years old. As his mother was still living, this indicated a separated part of her consciousness, a mind fragment. Her possessive and overpowering love, along with her fear of inadequacy for raising a child, had caused her to fragment and attach herself to her tiny son while still alive. Many cases of mind fragment attachment are family related, usually involving a parent in this or a prior life.

In the classic description of spirit attachment or possession, the living person is possessed by the spirit of a deceased person. Here the situation was reversed: a deceased spirit possessed by a living person.

Strong ties of love can interfere with the normal transition into the Light. Overwhelming grief of those who remain can hold a newly deceased soul back from moving on. A grieving person may welcome the spirit of a dear departed one and later find the consequences unbearable.

An EB can be drawn to any weakened part of the body and yet move about within the physical form. Such a moving sensation can indicate the presence of an intrusive entity. An entity can attach to an alter personality in a person with multiple personality disorder.

The attached discarnate entity becomes a parasite in the mind and body of the living. It imposes its own mental, physical, and emotional problems from its own immediate past-life experience and exerts influence on thoughts, emotions, and behaviors. Additionally, it imposes unwanted physical symptoms. All this can be confusing and frightening to the host and family members. Such intrusion by a discarnate entity can interfere with any aspect of life of the unsuspecting host, even one's taste for alcohol, food, even clothing.

Roberta and Her Mother

Roberta was in her mid-forties. She was a successful real estate broker, a capable woman. She heard a lecture on this subject and wanted to be evaluated for entity attachments. It was an excellent decision. Her mother had died about ten years previously and had immediately attached to her daughter. My questions were directed alternately to Roberta and her mother. Each answered in Roberta's voice, and some of the revelations surprised Roberta. Subsequently, her mother agreed to release into the Light. Roberta was amazed at what had just happened and was introspective for a few minutes. Still musing on the experience, she described a sudden realization, "Half my wardrobe is my mother's taste in clothes. I never liked those colors." Changes had begun in Roberta's life.

Cheryl and Her Grandmother

Cheryl attended a lecture on spirit releasement therapy. After the lecture, she approached me and asked a question.

C.: "Can an attached entity leave?"

Dr. B.: "Yes, sometimes they can leave. Why do you ask?"

C.: "I know my grandmother was with me after her death a few years ago. I could hear her voice. She even told me how to make pie crust. But she hasn't been talking to me for the last month."

I suspected the grandmother hadn't left, and I asked gently:

Dr. B.: "Grandmother, are you here with Cheryl? Are you here right now?"

Abruptly, Cheryl began to cry; her body began to shake. In a soft voice she said:

C.: "Yes."

Dr. B.: "You haven't spoken with Cheryl for the last month, Grandmother. What happened?"

C.: "I knew she was coming here. I didn't want her to volunteer for this. I don't want to leave."

Cheryl had learned of the lecture only days before. Her grandmother knew more than a month in advance. After a brief conversation with her grandmother, which included the resolution of a past-life trauma that involved her marriage with Grandfather in the current incarnation, she and Cheryl bid a tearful farewell to each other, and she went into the Light.

Olivia and Her Father

Someone who dies hungry for food or in need of drugs often attaches to an unsuspecting host in order to fulfill that need.

Olivia was divorced and living with her mother; she gained nearly thirty pounds in one year. Her father had died at the beginning of the year, unable to recover from surgery for stomach cancer. He had been fed intravenously, and he died hungry. Olivia's mother had sensed his presence immediately following his death. Suddenly he seemed to have left. He had joined his daughter, and that is when she started to overeat. Initially, she did not realize the extent of the weight gain until her twin sister visited at Christmas, still slim and pretty. Her father's insatiable hunger had driven her to overeat.

Following death, the Earthbound soul maintains its personality structure, with all the idiosyncrasies, emotions, character traits, and attitudes it had when living, as well as physical needs such as for food, alcohol, and drugs. This is a remnant of human existence. As a newly deceased soul moves into the Light, this residue of personality remains as part of the deep memory, or the soul consciousness that is carried from lifetime to lifetime. However, when an EB attaches to a living person, it still acts as if it were alive, manifesting its personality, habits, addictions, and other needs through the unwitting host. A victim of this condition can be amnesic about episodes of complete takeover.

The attached entity (or entities—rarely is there just one) uses the energy of the host. A living person can have dozens, even hundreds, of attached entities, as these occupy no physical space. The host usually feels a drain of energy and may notice some clouding of thought. Chronic minor fatigue may be the most universal symptom of spirit attachment.

The host is usually unaware of the presence of attached EBs. An attachment can form anytime: before birth, anytime during a lifetime, and beyond death. Thoughts, desires, and behaviors of an attached entity are experienced as the person's own thoughts, desires, and behaviors. If the attachment begins in early years, these characteristics do not seem foreign because they have been present for a long time. If an EB joins prior to birth, an undesirable condition might seem to be congenital. Most people would prefer to believe this rather than accept the possibility of discarnate spirit influence and entity attachment.

An afflicted person may report hearing voices yet exhibit no other psychotic symptoms. It has been fashionable among New Age enthusiasts to attempt to channel some higher power who will use the voice of a willing person to speak "words of wisdom." Some use the terminology "for my highest good" when calling for a spirit to channel through them. In essence, this welcomes a discarnate entity, the host granting permission to be used.

The identifiers such as "master" and "teacher" and qualifiers such as "for my highest good," may be claimed by the malevolent entities as their own identifications, qualities, or attributes. They lie. Unfortunately, some opportunistic entities who respond to this invitation refuse to leave at the end of a channeling session.

Altering consciousness with alcohol or drugs, especially hallucinogens, loosens ego boundaries, opening the subconscious mind to infestation by discarnate beings. The same holds true for the use of strong analgesics and the anesthetic drugs necessary in surgery. A codeine tablet taken for relief of pain from a dental extraction can alter the consciousness sufficiently to allow entry.

Following death by drug overdose a newly deceased entity maintains a strong appetite for the drug. This hunger cannot be satisfied in the nonphysical realm, and the newly deceased EB may attach to someone who uses drugs to maintain the sensations of the habit. Many drug users are controlled by the attached spirit of a deceased drug addict. In some cases, such an entity can attach to someone who is drug-free and influence them to begin drug usage. In many such cases, these and other addictions can be eliminated through spirit releasement therapy (SRT).

The Rehab Center

For several months, I volunteered at a women's drug rehab center. Of the nineteen incarcerated women who had SRT sessions, fifteen discovered EB attachments. All but one of these entities had died of drug overdose and had attached to the women at ages ranging from two to forty, inducing the desire for drugs.

A person who dies from drug overdose can seek another body to continue to satisfy the terrible hunger. The person who becomes host to such an entity can suddenly crave drugs and begin using them, even when there is no prior history of substance abuse.

One inmate at this rehab center was a dealer but had never used. The street people called her a "profiteer." The entity was a saloon keeper and madam, catering to the cowboys on cattle drives and local ranch hands. She would urge them to drink at the bar, use some "loco weed," then go upstairs to visit the girls. The madam never used drugs or alcohol. This same behavior was imposed on the young woman in the rehabilitation center.

A year later, seven of the fifteen women had not used or even desired drugs. Several desired drugs but used less; some did not return their survey forms. One woman returned to the center and was very angry. She had not used drugs and was intent on never doing so again. At a party, she drank a glass of punch that had been laced with LSD. The probation officers took a urine sample the following morning, and she was taken into custody.

The recidivism rate for drug rehab is between 60 percent and 90 percent. In this small sample of drug abusers, the results were promising, though not conclusive.

Present life relationship problems can originate in a prior lifetime when the two people were together. Couples counseling can be more effective if past lives are explored; partners often find the same past-life experience and locate the source of the present conflict. This can be resolved in the prior setting such that the present life is then free of the conflict.

In couples counseling both these areas must be explored. Attached EBs can affect one or both individuals. An attached EB can influence the choice of marriage partners or the desire to have an extramarital affair. A newly attached entity who dislikes the partner can drive the couple to divorce, even when there was no problem prior to the attachment.

Sandy and Steve

When Sandy and Steve met, they bonded instantly. Yet she became distressed over his outbursts of anger. Steve had served as a medic in Vietnam and had suffered unwanted and violent anger since leaving the military. Sandy had experienced a meaningful SRT session a few months prior to their meeting and she wanted Steve to have a session to explore his anger.

They never wanted to be apart. They wanted to do a "soul merge" before coming into Earth life again, incarnated as one person. I didn't know how that was done, but I didn't argue. In the session, Steve discovered many attachments, including wounded GIs who had died in his arms and the spirits of Vietnamese children, women, and Vietcong.

Lee was an officer who had attached to Steve immediately following his death in combat during his third tour of duty. He liked this big, gentle medic and was very protective of him. It was his anger that lashed out whenever he thought someone challenged Steve.

Lee was a powerful killer, and had been since his first combat experience in the war. It seemed the newly deceased spirit of Sergeant Chung, a Cambodian officer who died in the firefight, had joined Lee at that time. Sergeant Chung carried several EBs of Chinese warriors, attached in nested layers. Lee was a formidable personality with all this extra warrior energy. Lee helped the other attached entities to leave before he was willing to go to the Light himself.

Several weeks after Steve's session, Sandy called to say that she and Steve were going to break off their relationship. The chemistry was gone. This great attraction had never existed between Steve and Sandy. It was Sandy and Lee all along and had nothing to do with Steve. Not ever.

Sexual Vulnerability

Gay or lesbian lifestyle is more openly tolerated than ever before in our society. Same-sex orientation and behavior are no longer considered mental illness by health professionals. However, some individuals who are homosexuals, transvestites (cross-dressing in the clothing of the opposite gender), or transsexual (changing sex through gender reassignment surgery) are deeply disturbed by their desires. Only about one third of those who want to change can be helped by psychotherapy.

Sexual orientation can be influenced by an entity of the opposite gender. If an attached Earthbound soul is the source of the desire and the person wants to change, spirit releasement therapy is the treatment of choice.

Men who want to become women through gender reassignment surgery often describe themselves as a "woman locked in a man's body." In clinical practice we have discovered this to be an accurate description of the condition. The spirit of a deceased female joins a male body, often at a young age, and the boy grows up with the attached female soul, longing to come out and live as a woman.

In a landmark case, an exorcism accomplished what was considered impossible. A young man had been in treatment with a psychiatrist for several years in order to prepare him emotionally for gender reassignment surgery. In general, psychotherapy is considered ineffective in reversing the gender dysphoria, the desire for the sex-change surgery. During the young man's visit to another physician, who happened to be a Christian, an exorcism was performed, and twenty-two entities, including the female responsible for the urge to live as a woman, were expelled. The young man's desire for the surgery and female lifestyle disappeared completely.[14]

The openness and surrender of individuals during sexual intercourse can allow the exchange of attached entities between two people. Violence during sexual abuse opens the way for intrusion by a dark force entity (DFE). In every case of sexual abuse, rape, incest, or molestation we have treated, we found, through remote work on the perpetrator through the client, DFE influence with the perpetrator, and DFEs transferred to the victim during the abuse. All of these DFEs can be released into the Light.

Other Causes

Any mental or physical condition, strong emotion, repressed negative feeling, or unconscious need can attract a discarnate entity with the same or similar condition, need, or feeling. Anger, rage, fear, sadness and grief, or guilt can attract entities with similar emotions.

Physical trauma from auto collision, accidental falls, beatings, or a blow to the head can render a person vulnerable to intrusive entities. Even physical intrusions such as surgery or blood transfusion can lead to an entity attachment.

A colleague reported this case. A male client discovered and released a mind fragment of a living person. Near the end of the session, the therapist noticed a neat scar just above the ankle on the inner side of one leg. When questioned about this, the client revealed he had undergone a complete blood replacement shortly after his birth due to an Rh blood factor incompatibility. A fragment of the mind of a blood donor had joined him with the transfusion.

The mental, emotional, and physical influence of an attached EB can alter the path of karmic options and learning opportunities for the host. It can disrupt any detail of the Lifescript, a term I use for the original road map of the life, that was developed, with the assistance of several guides or counselors, in the Planning Stage in the Light before incarnating.[15] Souls can mark specific ages as checkout points, possible times of death, along the Lifescript. There is always something to be learned at the time of death, both for the person who dies and for those left behind. An attached entity can hasten death or prolong life, thus interfering with any potential checkout point and the intended learning.

An attached EB may be present without producing noticeable symptoms. A spirit attachment can be benevolent in nature, self-serving, malevolent, or completely neutral. An attachment to a person may be random, even accidental. It can occur simply because of physical proximity to a dying person.

However, connection with an EB may be the purposeful choice of either the entity or the living human due to an emotional bond between them in this life or in a previous lifetime together. In about half the cases of spirit attachment discovered in clinical practice, some association can be found, some unfinished business between them.

Even if there is some prior interaction between the host and the attaching EB, spirit attachment only perpetuates the conflict with little possibility for resolution. However, it must be stated that every experience has the potential for learning of some kind.

Although it seems to be a violation of free will, spirit attachment does not require the permission of the host. This appears to refute the popular belief that each person is responsible for creating his or her reality; there are no victims. The apparent conflict stems from the definitions of permission and free will choice. Ignorance or denial of spirit interference is no defense against spirit attachment. Belief or disbelief about the existence of intrusive entities has no bearing on their reality or behavior.

Few people refuse permission to these nonphysical intruders. They simply pay no attention. Individuals have the right to deny intrusion by another being. With limited knowledge and distorted perceptions of the spirit world, many people leave themselves open, creating their own vulnerability as part of creating their own reality.

The condition of spirit possession or attachment does not involve Light beings. Spirit guides and guardian angels do not attach or use the energy of living humans. They are here to assist, not force an agenda on the person. They make no decisions for the person, nor do they attempt to control in any way.

In the Planning Stage in the Light, where opportunities and challenges for the coming life are organized and planned, neither Earthbound souls of the deceased nor any other types of attaching entities are present. Except in rare cases, entity attachment is not part of a planned Lifescript.

A colleague reported a case of spirit releasement in which the client was a neighbor and the attached EB had lived and died in the neighborhood. The entity stated flatly the releasement session was part of the Lifescripts of all three of them, organized when they were in the prelife Planning Stage. The client had been an entity attached to the living person, now the attached EB, in another lifetime, and the being who would become the therapist had volunteered to clear the situation in the present incarnation.

These situations and conditions that can lead to spirit attachment, as just narrated, are taken from my actual case files. It seems that most people are vulnerable to discarnate interference many times in the course of ordinary living. This does not mean that everyone in the world is possessed. The best defense against the spiritual intruders is awareness of the condition and strengthening the "spiritual immune system" as described in Appendix B. We are not helpless victims in the struggle with unseen influences.[16]

Mind Fragment of a Living Person

It is not unusual to discover a mind fragment of a living person with a client. It may first appear to be an attached Earthbound soul, yet it turns out to be a fragment that has split away from the body/mind of another person.[17]

The Terminated Pregnancy

A pregnancy may end in spontaneous abortion or through medical intervention, usually by the choice of the mother. It can be a difficult and painful choice, and many women suffer intense guilt and shame following the procedure, as well as a sense of loss.

However, the burden of choice is not the sole responsibility of the mother, though it usually feels that way. In the spiritual framework of regression therapy, the Lifescript of each soul includes its own opportunities in the upcoming incarnation. No one is responsible for the choices of another soul. This certainly applies to mother and child. There is always a learning, a spiritual lesson, in each interaction between beings. And always present is love, unconditional and nonjudgmental.

Many situations—for example, marriage, pregnancy, and termination of pregnancy—involve two or more beings and each has its own part in the plan. If each being is responsible for its experience and the details of the Lifescript, then blame, shame, guilt, and remorse are false. We serve each other by fulfilling our agreed part on the Lifescript.

Inspirational Possession and Influence

Frederic Thompson was apparently influenced by R. Swain Gifford, a prominent artist who died in 1905. They had only a brief acquaintance prior to Gifford's death. The following summer,

Thompson gave in to overwhelming urges to paint. The subjects of the paintings were unknown to Thompson, yet on investigation they were found to be similar to Gifford's, in particular one of Gifford's unfinished works. In this well-documented case of possession, more accurately described as overshadowing, Thompson assumed the artistic skill of the deceased artist.[18]

Matthew Manning went to boarding school at age fifteen. Prior to his leaving his father's home, there had been an outbreak of poltergeist activity. Furniture was moved and rearranged, sometimes tipped over; puddles of water appeared on the floor; there were scribblings on walls; faucets and lights turned on and off. In the boarding school he attended, beds moved in the dorms, writing again appeared on walls, kitchen utensils rained into the dorms from out of midair.[19] This ceased only when Matthew took up drawing instruments and began producing sketches, drawings, and paintings, purportedly from deceased masters.[20]

Brazilian psychologist and psychic Luis Antonio Gasparetto reputedly produces works of art in the trance state, allegedly transmitted by the spirits of the great painters. He can hold a brush in each hand and in the toes of each foot, and can produce four paintings, the style of the deceased artist easily recognizable, in less than an hour.[21]

As a child, Rosemary Brown believed she saw spirits around her family. At age seven, Franz Liszt began to appear. She studied piano for a year as a child and a year and a half as an adult. Under the direction of, and partial possession by, Liszt, she gave excellent performances of difficult piano compositions.

Pearl Curran produced more than four thousand pages of fine literary work over a period of twenty-four years. The spirit, who claimed to be Patience Worth, transmitted the work written in late Medieval English. Curran had little education and limited exposure to English literature.

Robert Louis Stevenson credited his "little people," or "brownies," as he called them, for much of his literary output.

These are examples of *inspirational possession.*[22] There is no indication that the "possessors" are Earthbound souls.

Can higher beings impart skills to living people? Is it possible for a more advanced spirit to manipulate or control the mind and body of a living person, creating art, prose, or music such as these people produced? Such questions surpass human understanding and are part of the mystery of consciousness.

Some people can go into a trance or altered state of consciousness and allow other personalities to speak, using their voices. The older term is "mediumship"; today it is usually termed "channeling."[23] In the early days of nineteenth-century Spiritualism, communication from the spirits of the deceased consisted of raps and knocking sounds. This spirit communication changed to direct voice contact through persons with mediumistic ability. Then as now, loved ones in the Light can bring messages of assurance or assistance for ones still living. When they assume the familiar identity, there is recognition without fear.

Nonhuman Entities
Dark Force Entities

Some attached entities claim that they have never been alive in human bodies. Hostility and arrogance mark the dark force entity, or DFE. This is the classic demon as described in religious literature. We have learned much about these beings and their interaction with humans. In lectures and classes, we seek to dispel the extensive superstition and myth surrounding this subject, and to ease or erase the irrational fears engendered by the religious literature on demon possession and exorcism.

The DFE has historically been labeled "demon." There has been speculation that a demon is a projection of the human shadow, the externalization of the darker side of our personalities, as described by Carl Jung.[24] In twenty years of clinical experience, I have witnessed little evidence of that correlation. DFEs are not the shadow.

Extraterrestrial or Otherworldly Being

It is not unusual for a client to discover an entity that is nonhuman and not demonic, according to our methods of identification and differential diagnosis. This is an extraterrestrial, an ET. The ETs appear to be highly intelligent beings who claim to be from "far away" and only visiting here on some kind of mission. Very few of these have ever been human on this planet. This is not the spirit of a deceased extraterrestrial, but an alien in its normal form: non-physical. It seems we can choose to explore life in many locations and various forms.

Spirit Releasement Therapy

The good news is that something can be done about the condition of discarnate interference and entity attachment. Spirit releasement therapy (SRT) is a clinical treatment for this ancient problem. SRT can be used to help those who are troubled by the various attached entities that plague humanity. The treatment also helps the lost Earthbound soul, the EB, to find its way into the Light where it belongs. The extraterrestrial or otherworldly being, the ET, is guided back to its own home or homeworld. The dark force entity, the DFE, is transformed and taken back to its appropriate place in the Light.

The following sections offer only a brief description of the steps of SRT. Therapists who offer SRT to clients must have specific and thorough training to complete the work safely, for their clients and themselves.

Discovery

In the first step of SRT we attempt to discover any and all attached discarnate entities. This is not difficult with the client in an altered state. An attached entity seems to lodge at the level of the subconscious mind. It can hear and respond to us through the client's voice.

As the client relates the details of a personal problem or conflict, emotions emerge along with physical sensation or posture connected with the emotion. The client's descriptive words are used by the therapist precisely as spoken, and the client is directed to describe the sensation and give words to the feelings. These are just a few examples:

"If that **tension in your stomach** had a shape, a size, what would that be?"

"If that **sadness and tightness in your heart** could speak, what would it say?"

"If that **pain in your head** wanted to speak, what would it say right out loud?"

By personifying the sensation or image and urging it to speak, such questions often uncover an attached entity, a verbal response from a subpersonality (soul fragment), or a present past-life traumatic memory. If a memory emerges, it might be a painful incident in this life such as a scraped knee or bumped head. The memory will nearly always connect with an earlier similar incident in a previous lifetime.

The response is often a surprise to the client. The word or phrase just "pops up," and most clients will give voice to the phrase. The following words and phrases are typical responses.

"Yes."

"No."

"Go away!"

"Leave me alone."

"You can't make me leave."

"Help me."

"Let me out."

"What do you want?"

"Don't bother me, I'm busy."

"I don't want to talk to you."

"She's mine."

"Fuck you."

Any one of these responses will open a dialogue with the attached being, whatever it is. The question can be repeated in several ways until a response pops up. The response can be a physical posture.

One client held her forearms out from her body, her palms facing each other, shoulder width apart. Her arms were shaking. She was crying and didn't know why. No images were coming. I posed the next question.

Dr. B.: "If you were holding something in your hands, what would that be?"

She burst out with a sob.

C.: "It's my baby. It's my baby. And he's dead."

This uncovered a painful memory of a past life in which she had lost her infant. With resolution of this past-life trauma, her unexplained anxiety in the present life was eased.

The conditional tense is used in questioning: "*If* you were . . ." "*If* you knew . . ." implies a condition, and the subconscious mind fills in that answer, drawn from the deeper levels of far memory. It is a very effective therapeutic technique.

Identification

The second step is to identify what type of entity is present. Specific identification, or differential diagnosis, is necessary in this process because each type of attachment requires a different releasement method.

The Earthbound spirit of a deceased human is the most common attachment. However, there are many other types of nonphysical beings (spirits of nonhuman beings, various disruptive entities, and extraterrestrial beings, nonphysical in their normal state) that interfere with living people. These types of attaching and interfering entities will be described in later chapters.

The first step in identification of the source of the response is to determine whether the "voice" is part of the client or something/someone else. This is the primary diagnostic question:

Dr. B.: "Are you part of [client's name] or **someone** or **something** else?"

A past-life character, a subpersonality, or an alter personality in a person with multiple personalities will state immediately that it is definitely a part of the person. If the voice identifies itself as a young part of the client, the focus is on inner child healing.[1]

An attached EB will usually tell it the way it is. The DFE will be hostile in its declaration of being something else. The ET will often be condescending in its firm statement that it is something else.

Focusing attention on an emotion connected with a physical sensation is effective in eliciting a response that leads to dialogue with an attached entity.

Dr. B.: "If that anger and tension in your arms and fists wanted to talk to me, what would it say?"

This question often provokes a belligerent entity who challenges my right to interfere. It simply can't remain hidden and silent. Of course, that is the intent: Dialogue with the attached entity is an essential part of treatment.

The phrases and descriptions a client uses to depict their problems or conflicts can offer a clue to a spirit attachment. Such statements as the following suggest the presence of another being:

"I was different after _____."

"Other people tell me I changed after _____."

This can refer to illness, surgery, accidents, vacation sites, moving into a new dwelling, any sort of change or significant event.

"We were hiking up this narrow mountain trail . . ."

As the client recounts a recent event, the pronoun "we" may be used when describing a solo experience. There may be a subconscious awareness of an entity, and this languaging—which comes from the subconscious—suggests its presence.

One may describe an awareness of other "people" living inside. A person may hear voices and have no other symptoms of psychosis. Feelings of an internal battle of some sort or a sense of being taken over by something may prompt words such as the following:

"Something just comes over me."

"I watched myself doing _____."

"Part of me wants to do one thing and part of me wants to do something else."

"It's like my anger just lashes out. It's like someone just steps in and takes over."

The meaning of such language seems clear, and an entity can usually be uncovered with a question similar to the following.

"I want to talk to the part that says 'we.'"

"To you, the one who felt different after surgery, what happened?"

"You, the angry one, what's your name?"

A client may describe internal dialogue or argument. Conflicting feelings or attitudes can signal the presence of an active entity. This is not a case of simply weighing the alternatives before making a decision about something, but deep internal struggle over intention and desire, even behavior.

One might abhor drug usage and at the same time seek a source of supply. One young man often felt the urge to go out in the evening in search of a homosexual encounter. He fought the urge, especially since he was married to an attractive and sensual woman. This behavior started a short time after the death of a favorite uncle. The uncle had been gay.

In such cases, it seems as if two tracks of emotion, desire, or behavior are running simultaneously. This can be enormously confusing. Usually there is an immediate response when I ask the following question:

"I call out to the part that likes drugs. I want to talk to the part that uses drugs."

Hostility and defensiveness and an emphatic refusal to leave are definite indications of an attached entity. If the one speaking gives an account of its own death and subsequent attachment to the client, this is the memory of a separate, attached EB, the Earthbound soul of a deceased human being. We invite conversation with the personality speaking. An EB has lost only its physical body and may not be aware of its own death.

A client may suspect the presence of an attached entity after reading or attending a lecture on these subjects. Some people who learn about the concept for the first time have an intense physical or emotional reaction to the information. Usually this is the reaction of the entity. Many clients are referred by other people who have enjoyed positive results from spirit releasement. Many of our clients schedule appointments specifically to explore for attachments.

From the description of the problems expressed, I may suspect the presence of an attached entity. If there is another consciousness present, it will quickly become evident. In these cases, the direct approach is used.

The client is urged to express any "pop-up" answer, the very first thing that comes to mind in response to the following questions:

"Is there another person here, is there someone else inside this body? Is there another here besides [client's name]?"

If there is any indication of an answer, such as "Yes," a sudden pain in some part of the body, or an emotional outburst from the client, we can assume we have made contact with an entity of some kind. The second step in the identification phase of the session includes the following questions:

"Have you ever been alive in your own human body? Have you ever been human in your own physical body?"

If the answer is "No," there is a specific line of questioning related to nonhuman entities, described in later chapters. If the answer is "Yes," I continue to gather information related to Earthbound human souls.

"Male or female?"

The reply is immediate.

"What's your name?"

The entity usually knows its name. If it has been dead more than four or five hundred years, it may have forgotten the name. Time is not the same in the spirit world, but this seems to have an effect on memory.

"How old are you?"

The answer comes right away, except for females who died in their middle to older years. Some of them seem to be reticent about giving their age. We are always sensitive to their feelings.

"What year is it for you?"

The EB is often emotionally stuck in its traumatic death experience. Time "stands still" for these traumatized entities. The date for them is the year they died. As we saw with Dan in chapter 1, they typically impose the physical and emotional pain of their death on the host, whether they died of a heart attack (chest pains), crushed skull (headaches), starvation (compulsive overeating), drug overdose (addictions), falling (phobia of heights), drowning (phobia of water), or whatever else. The recurrent physical symptoms of the client may well be related to the death trauma of an attached entity.

Definitive answers to these questions will identify human entities: the Earthbound souls of the deceased, terminated pregnancies, or mind fragments of living people. When the answers are sparse or evasive, other diagnostic information is needed. Clear answers to the appropriate questions lead to correct identification. We continue to dialogue with the entity. Once the first one is identified, other entities also will want to interact with us.

Dialogue

The third step is dialogue with the entity to determine why and how it came to the client, circumstances that led to the attachment, the vulnerability or susceptibility that first allowed the entity to attach, its motivation for joining, and its effects on the host.

The entity will furnish information about the attraction and attachment through the following information-gathering questions:

"What attracted you to her?"

"Was it mutual in any way?"

"Did she invite you to come in?"

"Did she give you permission to join?"

"What was the opening that allowed you to get in?"

"How was she vulnerable to you?"

"How was she susceptible to you?"

The answers are often surprisingly honest and clear. This information is used in ongoing therapy to seal the leak, so to speak, preventing future spirit attachments.

"What was the purpose for attaching this time?"

"How does it serve you to be here like this?"

"Like this" refers specifically to the entity-human attachment. The spirit of a husband may have definite reasons for being with his wife. The spirit of a mother may feel she must stay with the child.

The drug addict may seek to experience drugs through the senses of the host. However, the desired effect cannot be fulfilled by attaching to a living human.

"How many lifetimes, including the present time, have you been with her like this?"

"Have you known this one [the client] in another lifetime when you both lived in your own physical bodies?"

If there was a past life together, the EB is encouraged to recall and describe the shared experience. The client will also perceive the lifetime recalled by the entity. In effect, it is a dual regression and can bring healing for both. The unfinished business that connected the two can be resolved, and release can be completed.

"Recall the last day you were in your own physical body in the lifetime when you knew each other. What happened?"

The death and separation of loved ones will be recalled with all the sadness and loss of that separation. The client and attached entity can be reassured that only the physical body dies. Love is forever.

The deathbed promises may be affecting the entity.

"I'll always love you."

This is the truth.

"We will be together again."

This is a loving promise.

"I'll never leave you."

An unwise and impossible promise, it often leads to spirit attachment.

Next, we explore the nature and extent of the interference caused by the attachment.

"How have you affected him/her physically?"

"How have you affected him/her mentally?"

"How have you affected him/her emotionally?"

"How have you affected him/her spiritually?"

"What damage have you caused him/her by being here?"

The responses to these questions answer many questions for the client. People take responsibility for their actions, and it eases their mind to know there was outside influence. It is important to note that in my twenty years of practice, no client has sloughed off personal responsibility and placed blame on an attached entity—an inspiring demonstration of personal integrity and responsibility.

Release

The fourth step is the actual release of the attached entity into the Light. The entity is instructed to focus upward and describe whatever it perceives. It often describes a brightness, a brilliant Light. The entity is usually greeted by the spirits of family or friends who have already gone on to the Light. Most often the one who comes is mother. For men who died in combat, it is more often their war buddies.

In the release process, the guiding spirits who come extend their "hands" to help the entity cross into the Light. Once this connection is made, the entity can be released from the client without fear of getting lost again or returning to the client. There is often a tearful reunion as the spirits of deceased loved ones welcome the Earthbound soul home. If one parent is attached to the client and the other deceased parent comes in the Light to lead that Earthbound parent home, the client can communicate with the one in the Light, perhaps for the first time in many years.

Sealing Light Meditation

The fifth step is a specific guided imagery of Light, called the Sealing Light Meditation.[2] It is important and necessary to metaphorically fill the space left by the departing entities. The client is guided to imagine a brilliant spark of Light deep in the center, to imagine the light glowing and expanding to fill the body, then expanding outward about an arm's length all around. It forms a shimmering protective bubble of Light surrounding the person. The client silently repeats this visualization several times each day. It is like a spiritual bandage over a spiritual wound.

Ongoing Therapy

The sixth step involves ongoing therapy. It is essential to resolve the conflict and to heal the emotional vulnerability that first allowed the spirit attachment. Inner child healing is helpful at this point.

Even though the condition caused by the attached entity seems to be resolved after release, there sometimes remains an impress of the habit, condition, or behavior—a sort of groove worn into the psyche. This remnant is more easily treated through traditional psychotherapy once the attached discarnates no longer burden the host. There are often additional entities discovered and released in further sessions. There is a sort of "layering" of attachments. Some clients seem to carry hundreds of these attached entities. A few have been burdened with thousands.

My Initiation

My initiation into this work came the first time I helped to free a lost Earthbound soul. I attended a meeting with a small group of people studying the phenomenon of channeling. The group leader channeled what seemed to be spirit teachers.

The focus for the group discussion was the choice for our life's work. The spirit control speaking through the leader asked each of us to describe that choice. When my turn came I shared my interest in spirit attachment and releasement. The control immediately announced that there was a lost soul in the vicinity and offered me a chance to put my words into action. It was a matter of put up or shut up. It sounded great, but though I had been studying and reading extensively on the subject, I had never actually tried it. I was very nervous. I was afraid of embarrassing myself, but I had to try something.

The Earthbound spirit spoke through the channel very clearly. In spite of my shaky effort, the process worked, and the spirit was eager to move into the Light when she saw it. It took about ten minutes. Another man in the group had a strong and unexpected emotional reaction to the procedure. He revealed that this was the spirit of his deceased wife who had died of cancer only months before. He was relieved to know she was safely on her path. Greatly relieved that the process had worked, I was also deeply moved by the experience. It was a sacred moment for me. It was my initiation into the work.

Within six months of starting my past-life regression therapy practice, more than half of my clients showed signs and symptoms of the condition traditionally termed spirit possession. I coined the term "spirit attachment" to better describe *interference* by discarnate entities. Although I couldn't see them, most of my clients could. However, I could talk with them through the voices of the clients. Within a few years, it became overwhelmingly clear to me that nearly everyone is influenced at some time, to some degree, for varying time periods.[3]

Over time I developed the techniques of spirit releasement therapy, largely by trial and error. Much of the technique I learned during sessions. An idea would pop into my head in response to a situation, and I would try it. If it worked, I would use it again on the next client. After reading something on the subject, I would try it out. If it worked, fine. If not, I would change it until it did.

After seeing the results of thousands of sessions, and reading and hearing accounts from other therapist's success with the methods, I am convinced that past-life trauma and spirit interference are the primary causes in many cases of mental and physical illness.

In 1980, I wanted to do a personal regression session with a past-life therapist in an attempt to discover the source of my own low back pain, which was interfering with my dental practice.

During my session, I discovered an attached entity. Airman Bruce was shot down over the Pacific in 1944; his back was broken during the watery crash. He spent some time in his emergency life raft, then drowned as his raft was overturned in heavy seas.

As a nine-year-old just after World War II, I was playing in the ocean with a war-surplus one-man life raft my dad had given me, the kind aviators carried in their fighter planes. The raft turned over. For a few moments, I felt helpless and a little panicky. Suddenly I felt very calm and safe, knowing I would be rescued soon, which I was. Airman Bruce had joined me; my situation was very similar to his. He meant to help. He was glad to go to the Light when he was shown the way.

However, his presence over thirty-four years may have led to some physical damage to several of my vertebral discs. The situation had bothered me for years, and there was no logical explanation or physical reason for the condition, which eventually forced me to leave my profession. In September 1982, I left dentistry on permanent disability with spinal disk degeneration. Even though I was physically limited, this was an important and positive change of direction in my life.

I went into a doctoral program in psychology, which I completed in 1988, earning a Ph.D. with a dissertation entitled, *Diagnosis and Treatment of the Spirit Possession Syndrome.*[4] It was the first ever dissertation on the clinical treatment of the condition, and I expanded the work into my book, *Spirit Releasement Therapy: A Technique Manual,* published in 1993.[5] I devoted my time to the study of psychology, past-life therapy, and the continuing development of spirit releasement therapy as the treatment for the condition of spirit possession, or spirit attachment. My life work had begun.

– 3 –

The Spirit of the Unborn

The Terminated Pregnancy

Though most souls of terminated pregnancies go to the Light, those who don't find the Light usually stay with the mother. However, they might attach to the next fetus when the mother becomes pregnant again. It is not unusual for a new baby to be born with an attached spirit of a would-have-been sibling. Some are discovered with other family members, some with people outside the family with no connection whatsoever to the family.

A thirty-something woman was urged by her boyfriend to have a session with us. He had seen some unusual, unexplainable attitudes and behaviors in her, and insisted that she schedule a session. She was not very cooperative and more than a little skeptical at the beginning of the session, but relented and agreed to participate fully in the process. She discovered the attached soul of a tiny infant. She had never been pregnant or married, and was in no way seeking such a situation at this point in her life.

During the session, she worked very well and the attached entity was released into the Light. After coming out of the altered state, she was still skeptical, somewhat incredulous, a bit embarrassed, and in a hurry to leave the office. Her boyfriend called a week later. On the weekend following her appointment, they were talking about the session. She suddenly burst into tears and experienced profound grief over the "lost" child. At a subconscious level, she was aware of the baby and felt the loss. Her session produced an unexpected healing for a problem beyond her conscious awareness.

The spirit of the unborn child presents a poignant situation in counseling, and these entities require special attention and careful explanation. They never had the chance to be born, to mature, to live life. In the Planning Stage in the Light they developed a Lifescript with several checkout points, including a prebirth termination. Even so, the plight of the helpless infant or fetus tugs at the heartstrings.

Since the legalization of abortion with the 1973 Supreme Court decision on Roe v. Wade,[1] the number of legal abortions has escalated enormously. As a result, we find many attached souls of aborted pregnancies.

Ideally, most newly deceased souls of people of all ages go home to the Light. However, many lives end at some point during the nine months of gestation, both from natural causes and induced termination. The incoming soul perceives itself as helpless and vulnerable and is confused about losing its body.

Pregnancy may terminate in a number of ways: miscarriage, either natural or as the result of an accident or trauma; intrauterine death; abortion; stillbirth; or the death of the mother. A being may leave the Planning Stage and linger in the vicinity of the future mother for a considerable period of time prior to conception, even several years. If the mother's body is destroyed in any manner, that being must return to the Light as part of the normal reincarnation cycle, just as any newly deceased soul must do. If it remains in the Earth plane, it is an Earthbound soul of an unborn human being.

A female client described her near-death experience during childbirth. It involved not only her but her baby girl, who actually died during delivery. After a difficult labor, the woman felt herself lifting from her body, free of pain. The soul of her baby girl rose beside her. She appeared to be about three years old. They lifted effortlessly, hand in hand toward a brilliant Light. The feeling of love between them was intense. At the entrance to the garden just outside the Light, her child, who now appeared to be about six years of age, turned to face her. Releasing her mother's hand, she held up her own precious little hand in a gesture meant to block her mother's further progress toward the Light.

In a clear, soft voice the child said, "You go back, Mother, it's not your time yet. I have to go now."

The woman reported that she felt such a complete exchange of love with her child during the experience, she never felt the need to grieve. Perhaps the total communication of love between the two fulfilled their mutual life purpose.

During the discovery phase of a session, an attached entity is sometimes found that has been human, and has no name or age but knows its gender. This information suggests a terminated pregnancy. The next question has to do with being born.

"Have you been born in your own human body?"

The answer is immediate.

"No."

This soul has no experience of being born. It has no name, and it is unsure if it even had its own human body, as it spent little time in the forming fetus. It often describes the body as "quitting" or "stopping," a naive way of describing death. This is the soul of a terminated fetus. Such discovery makes for a traumatic session and usually stirs up a lot of emotion for the client if she is the one who lost or aborted the child.

When offered the chance, the soul will make up a name for itself. It may be a descriptive term like "Sunshine," "Joyful," "White Cloud," or a common name like "Jim" or "Mary."

The soul is often very sad and cannot understand why its mother did this. There may be anger over the abortion. The spirit of the terminated pregnancy may attach to the mother because of anger and lack of understanding or simply the need for closeness. It may remain because it agreed to be a friend to the mother, not realizing the impossibility of friendship as an attached entity.

The spirit of the aborted fetus that attaches to the next viable fetus carries the traumatic memories of its own termination. As an adult, the host may have symptoms associated with memories of an abortion. The trauma, however, belongs to the attached entity. Release of the attached spirit of the terminated fetus erases the problem.

Twins

In some cases of twins, one fetus may die early in the pregnancy. The fetal tissue is resorbed and assimilated into the mother's body. All traces of that pregnancy disappear. The spirit of the deceased twin may then attach to the surviving twin, adamantly claiming that body as its own. The attached soul will experience the live birth, claiming it was, indeed, born.

The soul of the deceased fetus will be defiant, angry at the host, and insistent on staying. This is not an option. Further probing will reveal that there were two embryos and two waiting souls at the beginning of the pregnancy. The attached soul will tell the truth about going into the other following the end of its own forming body.

A brief explanation is frequently all that is required to resolve the conflict. A scan of past-life connections and an exploration of the Planning Stage and checkout points helps to ease anger, diminish pain, and bring understanding. The entity will change from the character of infant to a fully aware being. Usually they are eager to return to the Light so they can begin again. They deserve another chance and often get one very soon.

The Review Stage, the Great Halls of Learning, and the Planning Stage are known as important locations in the Light, like Union Station or Grand Central Station. Details of the coming life, such as choice of parents, relationships, marriage, geographical location to live, job or career path, potential checkout points—that is, death—are details of the Lifescript, the overall blueprint for the coming lifetime. In my model, this is how I have chosen to present it.

Patty and Her Brother

Patty, a thirty-eight-year-old woman, attended a group session. During a breathing exercise she developed a pain in her left side. While exploring this, she discovered an attached entity that identified itself as her would-have-been brother who died prior to Patty's conception. The mother was pregnant for twelve months; she had no menses for that length of time. The attending physician could not explain the condition.

The first fetus, the brother, apparently terminated naturally at two and a half months. He was extremely angry about the spontaneous abortion. Patty was conceived at the next ovulation. In its insistence to be born, the spirit of the terminated fetus attached to the new fetus immediately. Even in the face of this anger, I asked the question:

"Was there already someone there when you joined?"

The spirit acknowledged that there was another consciousness in the forming fetus, yet adamantly, though mistakenly, insisted that the new body was rightfully its own. Patty was the intruder.

This angry and confused soul was guided through past lives with his sister. He explored some of his choices in the Planning Stage prior to his brief physical existence. This finally dispelled the unwarranted anger. Forgiving Patty was the final step before he returned to the Light.

Abortion

An entity may attach to someone performing or assisting with an abortion. One female client remained with her adult daughter to comfort her during an abortion. The spirit of the terminated fetus attached to its grandmother. In a scan of past lives it was revealed that she was supposed to have been its mother in a former lifetime, and she had aborted it then. It had attempted to return to the family in this generation.

A nurse who assisted in performing abortions discovered that she carried over two hundred of these souls. Her compassion had opened the doors for them. She had to leave the job.

A forty-two-year-old woman discovered and released the spirit of a terminated pregnancy. She was six years old when it attached. Her father had been an abortionist, and his clinic adjoined their house. The spirit of the fetus, which had been six months along in utero, had a strong desire to live. The little girl next door was the closest living body.

Janet and Her Babies

Janet was accompanied to the session by her therapist. The progress of regular therapy had come to a full stop. At the beginning of the session, one question came to mind, and I asked:

Dr. B.: "Have you ever had any abortions?"

The woman practically shouted the words, surprised and overwhelmed by her sudden emotions.

C.: "Yes, I've had seven."

She clutched her abdomen, cried out in pain, and fell from the couch to the floor, where she remained for the rest of the session. She lived with a man, had no intention of marrying him, and had become pregnant seven times in as many years. She had chosen to abort every time. All seven souls of the unborn were with her, causing emotional pain and physical symptoms. They all claimed to love her and had chosen to be born to be her friend. They were frustrated at the impossibility of the situation. One by one they agreed to leave.

By the end of the session, Janet was free of pain, sitting on the floor and leaning against the couch. Later reports from her therapist indicated that their work progressed well after that highly emotional session.

– 4 –
Fragmentation of Consciousness

William James, the father of American psychology, wrote there was "much alarmist writing in psychopathy about degeneration," and he suggested that "if there are devils, if there are supernormal powers, it is through the cracked and fragmented self that they enter."[1]

Some attached entities claim to be human, to be alive in their own bodies and aware of the current date. They are not fixated in death trauma because they haven't died. These entities are mind fragments of living people, attached to other living people.

Multiple personality disorder was considered rare in earlier decades, if not fictitious. Mental health professionals have been extremely skeptical about the diagnosis. In recent years, though, this disorder has been identified as a valid mental condition with specific causative factors, with typical progression of the disorder, that can be treated with some success.

A number of autobiographies have been written by individuals who suffered childhood sexual trauma and developed many personalities or mind fragments as a defense. Some describe the experience of separating from their body and observing the molestation.

One woman recalled standing in the opposite corner as her grandfather fondled her while she was sitting on the toilet. Others describe watching from a place near the ceiling. One client described going out the window and sitting on the roof while her father did whatever he did to her little body lying in bed. When he left her room, she returned to her body.

Out-of-body experience is not unusual as the result of sexual abuse. Splitting, or fragmenting, and leaving seems to be part of the coping mechanism of dissociation. However, some of the "parts" do not return to the body/mind space. This can cause serious problems for the person who fragments in this way.

Even minor trauma can cause fragmentation. Who among us has not experienced some real or imagined physical, mental, or emotional trauma? During painful events in childhood, adolescence, even adulthood, mind fragments can separate from the main personality. These fragments can remain outside the body/mind space and refuse to return. With such parts missing, a person cannot operate fully in life.

This is the condition we have termed "soul fragmentation." In this condition, the terms "mind," "personality," and "soul fragment" are similar in meaning. Soul fragment, however, seems more accurate. Soul fragmentation can be discovered by the client in previous lives; a person can come into this life with part of the soul essence already missing, left behind in a traumatic event during a prior lifetime. Soul fragments can be attached to another person through several lifetimes.

People describe the condition of soul fragmentation in the following ways:

"all broken up"

"shattered"

"falling apart"

"out to lunch"

"nobody home"

"not playing with a full deck"

"brokenhearted"

"he stole my heart"

"empty-headed"

"not firing on all cylinders"

"one foot in the grave"

"part of me says 'yes,' part of me says 'no'"

"need to get my head together"

"need to pull myself together"

"need to gather my thoughts"

By contrast, it is a compliment to describe a person as "having his stuff together" or being "a really together person."

These idioms may seem like slang, yet they are often clear metaphoric descriptions of problems by people who have suffered soul fragmentation. A client may describe and experience feeling spacey, ungrounded, disconnected, like they are not in their body, with parts of the body feeling numb, not all here. Eyes may appear vacant and lackluster. Senses may seem muffled. Short attention span and poor memory both in daily life and in a therapy session can indicate the condition of soul fragmentation.

A person may sleep a lot and feel apathetic toward life. Feelings of depression may result from soul fragmentation. The client might feel as if something is missing. Clients express feelings of emptiness, having no heart, having an empty tube inside, or having a huge hole in their heart. Some complain that former lovers stole their heart. These and other similar expressions may well indicate a collective unconscious awareness of the condition of soul fragmentation.

In counseling, most of these separated soul fragments can be located and recovered. People can recognize, recover, and integrate these inner selves. As a result, the fragmentation no longer interferes with the enjoyment of life.[2]

Recognition of minor "splits" in the average person gives mental health counselors an effective method of discovering and treating deeper issues that plague clients.[3] In my clinical practice, I apply this knowledge with virtually everyone.

The Inner Family

It may come as a surprise to discover there is an "inner family" as well as our outer family of relatives and in-laws. The inner family is made up of our selves, our inner "team" of persons, each with a specific job to perform in daily living. This team begins development when we are infants.

The Protector/Controller

In that vulnerable state when the newborn is completely dependent on others, the behavior of other people is critically important. Some primitive part of the infant consciousness recognizes that some control over the situation is necessary for survival. This recognition leads to the development of the protector/controller, the first of our inner selves. It can be quite demanding, and not pleasant for caretakers. As the individual matures, this protector/controller self can become an obnoxious personality trait.

The first one to be manipulated by the baby's protector/controller is the mother. She gives food on demand, changes diapers when needed, and can be controlled by whining and crying. Mother and infant quickly understand the language by which the infant can ensure survival. The protector/controller guards the infant's vulnerability. As the infant matures, the adult is not so vulnerable and does not need the constant intrusion of the protector/controller. It may, however, continue to impose its original purpose, to protect the child from others. As an adult, the protector/controller can interfere with intimacy between love partners.

The Pleaser

Usually it is more difficult to control the father. Historically, fathers leave the care of infants to the mother, though there is a growing change in this pattern. Most fathers spend much time away from home; children have limited contact with them. The child learns to please the father to receive attention. This pleaser self becomes effective in manipulating people by being sensitive to their needs, in the hope that they will serve its own needs. This doesn't always happen. When the pleaser self is allowed to control behavior, it may focus totally on other people and neglect the inner child altogether.

The Perfectionist

The perfectionist self attempts to do things right so it will appear acceptable to other people and thus avoid criticism. The perfectionist is concerned only with appearances, as is the pusher.

The Pusher

The pusher self drives us to complete goals, to be productive, to appear useful. Neither the pusher nor the perfectionist is in touch with consensus reality, only self-centered inner reality. Both interfere with close contact in personal relationships. The pusher also interferes with any kind of relaxation.

The Critic

The perfectionist opens the way to formation of the inner critic. The job of the critic self is to catch errors before anyone else does, berating us in the process. We can correct our mistakes and others will think we are perfect. If we are perfect, we do not displease anyone. The vulnerable inner child is again saved from outside threat to survival. It is also protected from the intimacy of meaningful human interaction.

The critic points out so many errors and infractions of the rules of the-way-we-*should*-be that our self-esteem suffers. We learn early in life the rules of home, family, society—the way we are expected to be. Some invisible model of behavior exists that we are supposed to emulate. The critic self is quick to point out how often we fail to meet the standards of behavior and do not live up to the perfection of that model. Self-esteem, self-image, and self-confidence are undermined. This certainly leads to feelings of inferiority.

The Disowned Selves

We also have disowned selves, those parts of us we deny as being too sensitive, too caring, too sneaky, too weak, too sexy, too showy, too good, too capable, too angry—characteristics we judge to be unacceptable. These disowned selves are often attributes we project onto other people. When we judge others, feel hate toward others, distrust others, or have other strong negative reactions toward individuals or groups, we are seeing direct representations of our disowned selves. On the other hand, if we emotionally overvalue someone else, they are also representations of our disowned selves.[4]

The Inner Children

Healing the inner child is a popular topic. Many books and seminars have been offered on the subject of the wounded inner self.[5] The term "inner child" is a popular description for "subpersonality," the psychological definition of mind fragment.

The term suggests a single "inner child." This is misleading. In the human condition, there are many inner children, or mind fragments, of various ages, including prebirth. A fragment can split off if the incoming soul recognizes that the parents, or unwed mother, is considering an abortion. If the soul perceives that the family it is coming into will cause physical and emotional difficulty for the infant, the gentle, sensitive part can split away while the tough part remains.

This sensitive part might remain outside the body/mind space entirely. Such a split actually allows the child to survive in the early years, as the tough part is in charge of life. Here is an example:

A male client in his late thirties realized he was unable to enjoy intimate relationships requiring sensitivity and responsiveness. He wanted to change this behavior pattern. The client had been born into a low-income family with several children. His youth was spent in a tough New York City neighborhood.

In our session, he discovered a prebirth split; his sensitive part chose not to be part of childhood, and it separated. With his stronger, more insensitive side in control, he effectively survived his family and social environment in childhood and adolescence. As an adult, he was successful in business, assertive to the point of aggressiveness, and was fully aware of his insensitivity. When discovered, the sensitive soul fragment was more than willing to take its rightful place within. He was delighted to feel again, to interact from that place of caring and compassion.

Subpersonalities

Other selves or parts of the typical inner family are called "subordinate personalities" or "subpersonalities" in psychological terminology. A subpersonality is defined as a structured constellation of attitudes, drives, habit patterns, and belief systems, organized in adaptation to the internal forces (needs and desires) and external environment (perceived abuse or neglect). More serious emotional and physical trauma can lead to a breakdown or dissociation of personality and the formation of multiple personalities.

Subpersonalities are similar to the "games" of transactional analysis, or the "complexes" of psychoanalysis. A subpersonality is considered to be a mental/emotional construct, with a specific focus, that is "split off" from the whole of the personality, usually at a young age as a result of some unmet basic need, drive, or emotional trauma. It is self-aware and remains at the age at which the trauma occurred, continuously seeking to fulfill the unmet need or protect itself from similar trauma. By definition, the classic inner child (or children) is a subpersonality.[6]

A typical inner conflict caused by two subpersonalities can go something like this:

"Oh, what a beautiful outfit. I want it. I'd look so good in that."

"But it's so expensive, we really can't afford it."

"Oh, it's worth it."

"You are always wanting something new."

"Wow, I'd really look sexy. He'd really like me in it."

"No, I won't get it; that is just too much money to spend."

"Oh, you're just too, too, responsible."

"And you are too, too frivolous."

This kind of inner conversation is taking place between subpersonalities: parts in conflict. The conflict can be about food, alcohol, drugs, making purchases, dating, partying, sex, or any decisions about life. Part of me wants to do this, part of me does not. If the tug-of-war is evenly matched, the frustration can be paralyzing. The person doesn't know what to do. If the practical side wins, there is satisfaction in doing the right thing, maybe even a little smugness. But the other part feels cheated. If the frivolous part prevails, the immediate gratification is followed by guilt and self-recrimination.

Many female clients complain that when they try to be friendly to men, the men come on to them sexually. Certainly that is a normal part of the social scene, but clients describe something quite different.

They would reach out to men as they did when they were children, innocently reaching out to father for his approval and love. As mentioned, many fathers are absent, either working long hours, separated or divorced from the family, or deceased. This leaves an empty place in the child. The child often blames herself for the loss of the father.

When the child realizes the father is not coming back, there can be a fragmentation. The fragment is a young girl subpersonality who continues to seek her father's love. It is the subpersonality who reaches out through the arms of the woman for the attention and affection of the man, a substitute for her father. Men see only the adult woman inviting closeness and they respond as an adult male to a welcoming female. When he reacts normally the woman may be deeply offended, even feel violated.

This causes confusion and rejection for the man, confusion and pain for the woman who is being controlled by her own subpersonality without knowing it. Neither person understands the mechanism, and both feel hurt and angry. The pleaser and critic are at work here. When the child grows up to womanhood, the split is still present, still blaming herself and trying to please daddy or any other man in her vicinity.

We all have such "parts" within the structure of our personality that affect our habits, desires, and behaviors. Behavior changes can range from mood shifts to damaging eating patterns to relationship problems to violent behavior.

Dissociative Identity Disorder

In cases of extreme physical, emotional, or sexual abuse during childhood years, dissociation can become complete, resulting in two or more separate and distinct personalities, labeled "alter personalities" or "alters." The alters "switch" as each recurrently takes full control of the individual's behavior. This condition is termed "dissociative identity disorder" (DID), formerly "multiple personality disorder" (MPD). Between 95 percent and 100 percent of diagnosed multiple personality cases have a history of childhood incest, torture, or other abuse.[7]

In the dissociation of DID, reality contact is maintained through either the central or primary personality or an alter personality. The split is said to be massive or molecular; that is, each alter personality is complete, or nearly so, with its own name, memory of its own history, and relatively distinct and integrated behavioral and interpersonal patterns.[8]

Each alter personality has its own psychophysiological profile, which may include pain response; handedness; ability to heal and rate of healing; response to any given medication; allergic reactions; eyeglass prescription; diseases such as diabetes, epilepsy, and arthritis, including swollen joints; appetites; and tastes in food and drugs.[9]

An alter may be the opposite gender. This can lead to crossdressing or transvestism, and transsexualism, the desire to undergo sex change surgery. An attached EB of the opposite gender can urge the same choices.

Dissociation is considered a coping mechanism for a traumatic or overwhelming stressful situation. Not all people who suffer this kind of abuse develop DID. It seems to depend on the innate capacity to dissociate in response to the posttraumatic stress of the abuse.[10]

Many health professionals refuse to accept the existence of multiple personalities. For this reason, many people are misdiagnosed by therapists. It has been shown that many cases are not diagnosed correctly for a period of more than six years.

However, the disorder is recognized by the American Psychiatric Association as a condition that affects an unknown number of people. Many women and some men with DID find a therapist who can help. Many men with the condition end up in prison due to violent behavior.

DID is a serious disorder, and it requires treatment. Some people with the condition function fairly well in society, but most have serious problems with work, marriage, and family. There is treatment for such a condition, though it usually takes several years for the successful fusion of the various alters.

DID and Spirit Releasement Therapy

An entity can attach to a specific alter personality. The attached entity will be associated with only that alter, and manifest at no other time, as we can see in the next case.

Julia was approaching her fortieth birthday. She recalled being raised in a transgenerational satanic cult. Her parents and their parents before them had worshiped the dark forces. As a child, Julia was sexually used and abused in the rituals of the cult. As a result of this deliberate torture, Julia developed multiple personalities and was diagnosed with DID.

This is not unusual in such situations. As an adult, she had escaped both her family and the cult. In therapy for her condition in another city, she was referred to us by her therapist, who was familiar with our work, to uncover and release the dark force entities associated with the cult activity.

There had been hypnotically embedded programming which decreed that she return to the cult at a future date, likely triggered by her fortieth birthday. Though she had thus far resisted the command, she was feeling the pull to return. During the session in which we were seeking the source and location of that command, the "Priestess" alter came out with a grimace and a growl. The behavior of this alter had frightened her therapist and was the motivation for referring Julia to us.

Priestess was in charge, she haughtily informed us, and she had allowed Julia to enter therapy for a short while. She deemed it harmless and no threat to herself or the cult. Soon she would come out and take over completely, then return home to assume command of the cult. The cult leaders had convinced her of her unique specialness. After all, she informed us, she had been trained for just such a role. She assured us there was nothing we could do for Julia.

Priestess was directed to recall the rituals in which other girls had been sexually used, just as she had been. She easily recalled such instances. We bluntly questioned her statements. She had been told secrets regarding her future role in the cult, and didn't she think the other girls were told the same secrets? With so many girls treated in the same way, did she think she was the only one to be singled out for this honor? Wouldn't they ensure their future leadership by creating many such priestesses? And tell them all how special they were? The cult leaders were not dumb, were they?

We continued pressing, intent on injecting doubt into her story. Julia had escaped, perhaps others had also escaped, perhaps some had died. She was obviously intelligent—did she think she was the only one? Maybe the cult leaders had lied to her. Maybe they didn't care about her, just about themselves and the continuation of the cult. What did she think of them now?

This line of questioning gave Priestess pause for a moment. Then she growled in anger and reaffirmed her specialness and stated that she was going back soon to take her rightful place and there was nothing we could do about that. This arrogance and ego inflation, along with the history of satanic cult ritual abuse, was a red flag indication of an attached DFE.

Dr. B.: "Priestess, look inside yourself. See if there is something or someone else controlling you as you control Julia. How would you feel if you were being controlled by something else? What if you were not so special or powerful as you think?"

This kind of challenge cannot go unanswered by an entity, a person, or an alter personality that is oppressed by demonic influence. In a huff, Priestess explored inside herself (whatever that means) and discovered a black blob. It had red eyes.

This was the dark force entity assigned to her to ensure compliance with the plan of the cult. So far Julia had resisted the commands. The DFE was released appropriately; it was glad to go. When they plug away at their job over time without success, continuously thwarted, DFEs tire, and often express weariness with their assigned task.

Dr. B.: "Priestess, how does that seem now? You were controlled by that thing they put there. How does it feel now that it's gone?"

C.: "It feels so strange. I'm not the Priestess anymore. I'm not going back to them. Not ever."

Dr. B.: "Would you like to take a new name?"

C.: "Yes, please give me a name."

Dr. B.: "That's for you to choose. You have the right to choose your own name."

Her voice was no longer angry or growling. She was quite soft and gentle, not subdued, but calm. This took her a few moments. There was no urgency now.

C.: "I will take the name Sarah."

Sarah was described in the Old Testament, the wife of Abraham and mother of Isaac, the progenitor of the Jewish people. Priestess had a commanding presence, her leadership abilities would have been put to foul use in the cult, had she returned. But now, the capability of this alter personality could be well utilized as she integrated with Julia. The work of this session was deeply satisfying to this woman. No longer would she have to fight the urge to return to the terribly destructive lifestyle of the satanic priestess.

Soul Fragmentation

Shamanism is an ancient form of spirituality and healing practiced in indigenous cultures around the world. Soul retrieval is a shamanic approach to healing. In the tradition of shamanism, illness is an indication that the soul has vacated the body. The shaman enters an altered state of consciousness through the rhythmic beating of a drum or by ingesting a plant substance such as peyote or ayahuasca. The shaman is able to journey into the upper world, the lower world, or wherever the soul is located, to retrieve the soul and return it to the sick person, restoring wholeness and health.[11]

In 1989, I heard a lecture on the work of Sandra Ingerman, as described in her book, *Soul Retrieval*. As the presenter described various forms of soul loss, it became clear to me that these conditions were a part of my practice that I had never recognized. Mind fragments of living people are sometimes discovered as attached entities, yet I hadn't considered the other person who had lost the fragment. I found confirmation of this type of attachment in Ralph Allison's book, *Minds in Many Pieces*, and Adam Crabtree's classic work, *Multiple Man*.

Alter and subpersonalities are the standard fragments; they remain within the person's body/mind at the subconscious level—except sometimes when they leave the premises. For the purpose of clarity in my own understanding and way of presenting the material, I describe several categories of fragmentation.

Submerging

This subpersonality or soul fragment is often discovered as the severely damaged inner child. Careful and sensitive work is required when dealing with the vulnerable inner child that has submerged.

Trust is a major issue. The adult client may deny the existence of this subpersonality. Its very existence is at first rejected by the only one who can understand its pain.

The initial stage of therapy involves the adult and is aimed at recognition and acknowledgment of the dysfunctional family, especially abusing parents. Failure to recognize and treat this submerged inner child may result in physical illness. The child is the foundation for a person's life, and this fragment of consciousness may have submerged as the result of past-life trauma.

Candace was a highly intelligent, efficient, well-grounded, no-nonsense businesswoman in her late thirties. She had engaged in a few romantic affairs but had never committed to a serious relationship. Then she met Rick, an affable, open-hearted Italian, and things quickly changed. Passion became part of her life, and she was seriously contemplating marriage.

Candace was troubled; in intimate moments she found herself becoming numb, almost mechanical with Rick and his affections. Planning her life with him, turning her affections toward him exclusively, and facing a full life ahead, Candace was puzzled by this behavior. She felt vaguely angry at some of his behavior and his inability to make sound judgments.

In past-life exploration for the source of the anger and numbness, she discovered a scene in which she saw herself holding his body and wailing loudly. He had lost his life in a senseless battle. It felt like part of her had just died inside. For the remainder of that life she was mechanical, devoid of emotion. It was safer; feeling was too painful.

Guided back to circumstances leading up to this trauma, Candace recalled a terrible argument the night before in that life. The argument was about his decision to engage in this battle. He had pledged himself militarily to the unscrupulous leader of their people, believing military duty to be more important than staying with his family. She did not share his loyalty to the leader. She knew the danger of the coming battle and considered his decision to be stupid. Although she knew he would not survive, she could not put this into words. He and many other peasants fought with pitchforks and clubs. They all died in the fields.

Candace scanned her present-life body. There was an emptiness and a huge hole in her heart. There was buried anger, deep sadness, and the familiar numbness. The fragment had submerged deep inside, becoming dormant, numb—almost dead.

Dr. B.: "Help her up. Help her like an old woman. Help her gently. Has she seen all this? Does she understand?"

C.: "I think so."

There was wonder and surprise on Candace's face.

Dr. B.: "What does she want from you?"

C.: "She wants me to voice the feelings. The things she couldn't say then."

Dr. B.: "What will she give you in return?"

C.: "Joy."

With a smile beginning to form, Candace deeply felt the transformation of sadness, anger, and feelings of numbness. This was the beginning of major change for Candace. As she later described it, "The walls came tumbling down."

Shifting

Among traumatized people, a common condition is feeling partially out of the body or not quite all the way in. The client may describe feeling "spacey" or "airheaded." In the session they may seem to drift away, and their attention span may fluctuate. This is a shifted fragment, slightly ajar in some direction, usually upward or sideways, sometimes back from the body.

Chandra, a forty-five-year-old female client, talked about herself in this manner. During one session, I felt that I should focus my eyes about four feet above her head to look at her. I asked where she was in her body. She described floating upward, her feet at about chest level. She had endured numerous surgeries and was allergic to many things, including some medications. Her father had begun molesting her at eighteen months. It started as fondling, but at age thirteen he actually penetrated her. This continued until she left home at eighteen to get married. She had not developed MPD as a coping mechanism; she had gone out-of-body to escape the abuse.

Fading

This is a typical behavior of children in dysfunctional families. They describe wanting to fade into the woodwork, to vanish into the furniture. Literally they try to disappear. They do not engage in life, and such behavior continues into adulthood. Such people may be quiet in a group. They dress plainly; women use little or no makeup. Others have difficulty recalling their presence. They just fade from one's awareness.

Melissa attended a three-day seminar. Plainly dressed, she wore no makeup. Her skin was pale, her thin hair a colorless blond. Participants arranged the chairs in a circle. Melissa moved her chair back from the circle. In a demonstration session on the second day, she revealed she had been living with a man for seven years but with no intention to ever marry. She discovered in the altered state that she had never committed to be in this life at the time of her birth. This happened before I learned about soul retrieval, and I had no knowledge of how to recover her soul essence. Melissa did not show up on the third day of the seminar.

Separation

The soul is connected to the physical body by the silver cord.[12] In the condition of fragmentation, each fragment maintains a connection with the core consciousness by a silver thread, a fiber of the silver cord. In separation fragmentation, a fragment leaves the body/mind, maintaining the silver thread connection, and it is this link that makes the recovery process possible.

The body can function as long as the silver cord maintains its connection, even if there is total evacuation of the fragments. In cases of total fragmentation and separation, the body is normally in coma, unless inhabited and controlled by a strong entity.

When the silver cord disconnects from the body at death, the fragments continue to be joined to each other by the silver threads, even after the being leaves the physical body. The soul fragment associated with a severed body part remains with the body part, yet is still connected by a thread to the main soul consciousness, wherever that is.

Severe trauma usually results in significant fragmentation of the soul essence. The fragment escapes and does not rejoin but follows at a safe distance, connected by the silver thread. This is the person who is "not at home," "not playing with a full deck," "out to lunch," or "empty-headed."

A person in this situation is vulnerable to spirit intrusion or possession. With such fragmentation, it is easy for another consciousness to enter, become established, and take some degree of control.

Separation fragmentation often happens following emotional trauma such as a "broken heart," depression and suicidal urges, explosive anger followed by guilt over the behavior, or physical trauma such as wartime combat, amputation, severe beating, incest, or rape.

Evacuation

A separated fragment can remain in the location of the past-life traumatic experience. This is considered evacuation; it is a fragment separated by time and distance. Terror can lead to fragmentation and evacuation, although the silver thread remains connected. A significant percentage of the soul essence can abandon the physical body and attach to another living person in the present life. A soldier might leave a major fragment in a battlefield. Severe depression can actually cause a fragment to move into the Light; a kind of "little death." Death of a loved one can bring about this condition.

People in a relationship often exchange fragments. The relationship can be male and female, parent and child, or any other close interaction. When one of the partners in such a relationship dies, and the newly deceased soul moves into the Light, attached fragments of the survivor are also carried there. Those fragments can be recovered and reintegrated with the survivor. However, these attached fragments with the survivor can act like a magnet to draw the newly deceased soul, causing an attachment.

Physical Mutilation

Decapitation as punishment had a terrifying history following the first use of the guillotine in 1792, ending in 1981 when capital punishment was abolished in France, where it was predominantly used. The device was invented by Dr. Anton Louis and named after Dr. Joseph Ignace Guillotin, a humanitarian physician who argued for a quicker and less painful death than the commoners suffered by rope or the nobility by sword.

In earlier times, battles were fought between warriors armed with swords. Heads rolled. Serious accidents can result in decapitation. Surgical removal of body parts—small as teeth or appendix, or large as arms or legs—might lead to fragmentation and separation of the fragment of consciousness associated with the body part. Some heart transplant recipients report feeling that someone is following them. Often it is the soul essence or a mind fragment of the organ donor. Other mind fragments can follow other organs, attaching to organ recipients.

Atrocities in wartime reveal the savage nature of men. In the male mind, a commonly held misperception is that genitals make the man. Throughout the history of war, soldiers have mutilated enemy casualties on the battlefield; genitals are severed and stuffed in the mouth. This was repeatedly seen in the Vietnam War. American dead were discovered in this condition. It is a supreme insult meant to discourage and intimidate. It works.

Fragment Recovery

Some soul fragments that separate during traumatic incidents do not return to the body/mind space. The fragment sometimes refuses to return for fear of repeated trauma. This leaves a void, an emptiness, a hole in the heart, or some other similar feeling that can be felt and described.

The client in an altered state is directed to scan the body. They may discover dark or shadowy spots, voids or holes, hollow tubes and empty places. These are the etheric spaces left by soul fragmentation. The client is directed to focus on these spaces, to look for threads that lead out from the empty place. These threads can be perceived by about half of all clients. The client is directed to choose the thread which seems to be most prominent and to follow that one. It will lead to a scene, an event, or trauma in this or another lifetime. The client will recall the event, observe and describe the trauma, and experience the splitting away of the fragment.

If the client does not find the threads leading outward, the focus shifts to the emotions and memories connected with that void or emptiness. This will usually uncover the traumatic event. For the nonvisual person, the emotions and physical sensations associated with the empty space emerge, and this will lead to the painful memory.

Exploration uncovers the circumstances leading to the event and the traumatic experience itself. The fragment, the subpersonality formed by the fragmentation, retains the mental, emotional, and physical residues of that trauma.

As the client recalls traumatic childhood events, the child at that age is seen and described. The young subpersonality must be shown that it survived the trauma, that it did not and will not die, and that this adult—the client—is who it became. The primary fear of the child during the trauma is that it will not survive.

After the traumatic event is processed to peaceful resolution, the conflict resolved, and the painful memories healed, the soul fragment is welcomed into the body wherever it belongs. The client is urged to visualize kneeling and reaching to the child part with open arms. In the imagery, the child almost always runs into the arms to be hugged. Like every piece of a jigsaw puzzle, the fragment is an important part of the whole.

Each soul fragment locates its perfect place in the puzzle as it enters the empty space, wherever that may be—sometimes the head, more often the heart. The client will describe feelings of warmth, being fuller, more whole.

The fragment always brings a gift when it returns. The gift can be a characteristic or ability, such as playfulness, creativity, spontaneity, fun. The clients as grownups who are recovering their soul fragments also have a gift for the fragment or fragments who return. It is usually described as love, safety, security, attention, and the willingness to listen to the little part now that it is home.

Invitation to Fragmentation

Tina and Annie

In a phone conversation with me, thirty-year-old Tina described a serious automobile accident involving her friend Annie, who sustained massive physical damage and was not expected to live. She clung to life and was suffering terrible pain. Tina visited her friend in the hospital and in her love and compassion, expressed her desire to help.

"Oh, I wish I could take some of your pain."

After that visit, Tina began to experience pain in the same areas where Annie had sustained wounds. I asked Tina to guess how much of Annie's essence had joined her. Quietly, she looked within and discovered that a 30 percent fragment of Annie's consciousness had come in. Apparently, Annie fragmented severely in the accident and had accepted Tina's invitation. Tina did not want to release the fragment for fear her friend would die, and she did not schedule a session.

Fragmentation and Depression

Cindy and Her Stepfather

At thirty, Cindy was barely functional in life. She was divorced, raising her five-year-old daughter alone. Cindy was depressed to the point of being suicidal. She was an incest survivor and had been working on that issue in therapy. Her deceased stepfather had been the perpetrator. It is not unusual for a deceased perpetrator to become an attached entity. Guilt surrounding the incest is the impetus for attachment to the child in an attempt to seek forgiveness. However, there was something else involved in this case.

As Cindy recalled the incest she described fragmenting and separating, and estimated the fragmentation at about 60 percent. When the separated fragment was discovered, it was a six-year-old subpersonality—Cindy's age when the incest happened. It had remained separated from her since the time of the molestation. The fragment was invited to rejoin Cindy but adamantly refused. When asked why she rejected the invitation, she reported that the stepfather was still there, clearly visible to the separated subpersonality, and she was afraid to come any closer. She agreed to remain nearby and observe.

Cindy was directed to recall her stepfather's face as best she could. She immediately had the image, and described his face as alternating between human and animal—a wolf with red eyes. Attention was then focused on the attached entity. Through years of doing this therapy, we have found that in every case of sexual violation the perpetrator is

always influenced by an attached DFE. The stepfather was belligerent at first, claiming ownership of the woman and the right to do
with her as he pleased. This is a strong indication of the presence of
a DFE.

His words indicated confusion, lack of understanding regarding
his behavior, and at the same time, he expressed love for his step-
daughter. With further probing into the cause of his actions, he
recalled that his mother had touched him, had hurt him when he
was about two. At the time of that incest, his anger, fear, and pain
opened the way to DFE infestation which transferred to him from
his mother. It was still with him.

He was directed to look within himself. He discovered the DFE
that had caused distortion of his thinking while he was alive and was
still distorting his thinking. It was released appropriately. As this
interference was removed, his distorted thinking was cleared, and
he was immediately remorseful and apologetic.

Communication between stepfather and daughter at this time
began to relieve the woman's anger and hurt and the stepfather's
overwhelming guilt. When Cindy's fragmented subpersonality was
finally willing to forgive the man who violated her as a child, he also
was willing to forgive himself. Then he could be released into the
Light. Only after he was gone was it safe for the young fragment to
return and integrate with the client. Cindy's condition began to
improve immediately.

Fragmentation and Past-Life Therapy

Recovery of soul fragmentation is an important approach to
healing. In many cases the fragmentation occurred in a past-life
traumatic incident. Past-life therapy techniques are used to resolve
the mental, emotional, and physical residues, and the integration is
accomplished in the past-life setting. The client can usually feel the
difference immediately.

The Musicians

A female client discovered that a fragment of herself in another
life had attached to her lover in that time. He was a piano player in

a honky-tonk bar, and she was his singer. In the present life, they were again lovers, and both were musicians. Her fragment from the other lifetime had separated from him and had remained Earthbound after his death. The fragment had found him again in the present lifetime and had reattached. This is not unusual for an Earthbound entity.

In the session, the fragment was separated and sent back to her character in the past life, the emotional issues were resolved, and the past-life personality was moved into the time of her death. Once in the Light, the being was moved to the Planning Stage for the present life, moved into the infant body, then forward in time to the present moment, reuniting with the client.

Some sub- and alter personalities claim to have been the primary manifesting personalities in a past life of the client. The alter might have emerged in the present time to assist the present personality in coping with an unbearable situation.

Connie and Her Protector

At forty-two, Connie was a marriage and family counselor. She had begun studying psychology at age thirty-two. Only three years prior to her session, she had discovered in the course of her own therapy that she had been molested as a child. From age three until age ten, her father had sexually abused her. At ten, a twenty-two-year-old male alter personality emerged. This one stood up to the father and just said, "No more." Apparently this alter had enough authority to persuade the father to cease the abuse.

Connie was already working on the inner child subpersonalities with her own therapist. In our session, several entities were released before the twenty-two-year-old male emerged. He was certain he was not a separate entity but part of her soul consciousness, claiming to be the manifesting personality in a former lifetime. He was called up from dormancy in the unconsciousness as the result of her stress and pain caused by the molestation. He was not treated as an attached spirit, and he was not integrated in this session. Connie did not return for further sessions.

Jessica's Heartbreak

If a fragment has split off from a past-life personality in a traumatic episode and remains there, it cannot simply be brought back directly into present time and integrated. The fragment is part of the past-life personality and is still Earthbound, similar to the newly deceased spirit that does not go to the Light after death, but remains Earthbound.

Jessica recalled a love affair during a vacation in France a decade before. She fell in love, only to be hurt, as circumstances prevented the affair from maturing. A fragment of her "heart" remained in the romanticized setting, and sadness was the emotional energy maintaining fragmentation. Exploration uncovered a passionate love affair in France in a past life. She had met her lover in a secluded garden, expecting romance and even a proposal of marriage. Instead, he broke off the affair; she was devastated.

She was heartbroken, and that fragment remained floating in the garden, dazed from the trauma. As a result, Jessica was born into this life in a fragmented condition. The past-life fragment was guided to understand what had happened and was finally willing to rejoin the young woman in that life. She was then guided forward to her death and into the Light, and finally into the present life, where she took her rightful place as part of Jessica.

Her recent painful love affair had brought her into therapy, where she discovered a similar event in another time. Both fragments were reunited and integrated. It frequently happens that a present-life event echoes a past-life trauma, and in such cases both can be healed.

The Chocolate Chip Cookie Eater

In some cases, the fragment splits off from the core personality in a present-life traumatic event that is similar to the death trauma in a former lifetime. The fragment can easily recall the lifetime and the circumstances that led to death in the earlier time. Past-life therapy techniques can help lead to integration of these fragments.

Some years ago, I attended a workshop on healing subpersonalities. We were instructed how to discover one of our own subpersonalities, to recall the trauma that caused the split, to determine what need or desire was denied or thwarted, how it affected us, and how to resolve it. Mine turned out to be "CCCE," the Chocolate Chip Cookie Eater.

When I was about nine years old, my folks left me with a favorite aunt for the weekend. She had no children and she doted on me. She made me chocolate chip cookies. She transferred them from the cookie sheet onto a plate while they were still warm. The smell was tempting, and I reached for a cookie. She slapped my wrist. I couldn't understand why she did that. Again, I reached for a cookie. Again, she slapped my wrist and told me I couldn't have a cookie.

Then I got it! No cookies! She had made them for me and now she was keeping them from me. I was confused! She was being mean to me and I was hungry and they would taste so good. My mouth was watering and I could almost taste the warm soft chocolate chips and now I couldn't have them. Of course I wanted them even more, but she had some strange idea that the cookies had to cool before I could have one. So near but yet so far.

Unsatisfied hunger, thwarted desire for the sweet cookie, and the abrupt withdrawal of my aunt's love were all too traumatic for my young mind. Such are the conditions that lead to the formation of a subpersonality. My Chocolate Chip Cookie Eater split off. The CCCE was born, and its job was to acquire and consume chocolate chip cookies. It did its job well.

Since that time, chocolate chip cookies have always been my favorite. When Mrs. Fields cookie shops opened across the country, I was delighted. What a great taste, and they were so big. I could easily eat a half dozen with a cup of coffee. Expensive, but that mattered not one whit. I would always buy a dozen, just in case.

The workshop leader then guided us in locating the origin of our subpersonality. As I allowed my subconscious mind to locate the cause of the split, I discovered a past-life memory of myself as an eight- or nine-year-old boy, youngest of a large family in extremely poor and primitive circumstances. There was not enough food for everyone. We ate at a rough wooden table with bench-like seats. My siblings were harsh and mean to me. I recalled being shoved off the end of the bench often, and watching them take my food. Eventually I died of malnutrition.

When my aunt slapped my wrist and prevented me from having "my" cookies, that memory was triggered in the subconscious mind, below conscious awareness. The split was formed and that fragment had to make sure I didn't starve again. This time the focus was chocolate chip cookies. With past-life therapy on this traumatic life and death from malnutrition, the split was healed. I still enjoy chocolate chip cookies, but I am not a driven man. I seldom buy a dozen at a time.

Clients feel the past-life resolution and integration of the fragment as a warmth, a fullness where there had been a void. Past-life therapy is completed on a subpersonality which was fragmented and separated in another lifetime. The subpersonality is integrated in the earlier time frame and the soul is brought through the Light into the present moment. Clients feel the result here and now. Recovery of soul fragmentation and past-life therapy are complementary techniques that are effectively used together.

Past-life therapy and recovery of soul fragmentation are complementary approaches to healing. In a session, the two methods weave together seamlessly, which is why this is an essential tool for the well-prepared therapist.

Fragmentation and Spirit Releasement Therapy

Psychiatrist Ralph Allison has described cases of apparent spirit possession affecting his clients diagnosed with dissociative identity disorder. In his conceptual scheme of this phenomenon, he includes the Earthbound soul of a deceased human, an aspect or fragment of the mind of a living person, and full demonic possession.

The practice of witchcraft and black magic, the casting of spells, hexes, and curses, for example, can cause fragmentation of the practitioner, witch, or sorcerer. It is significant that the fragment of consciousness gives energy to the curse. This fragment remains with the victim of the magic spell or curse. There are always dark force entities involved in this sort of intrusive activity.

Other clinical investigators have discovered mind fragments of living people attached to clients. Mind fragments of a living person can be attached to one or more other living persons. The condition of fragmentation is not healed by death of the fragmented person. This means that the newly deceased spirit, the discarnate entity, remains fragmented. This fragmented entity can then attach to still another living person. Thus, an entity can be attached to two or more living individuals.

In many cases the fragment comes from a close family member, a spouse, or a possessive and protective parent in this or a prior life, in particular the loving, overprotective, overbearing, and possessive mother.[13]

A loving, protective mother can fragment and attach to each of her children before and after death. Following her death, her fragmented soul can attach to any one of the children or can fragment further and split herself between her children. Each child may be carrying several soul fragments of mother. If this condition is discovered in session, all the fragments must be recovered before the entity is sent to the Light.

In practice it is not unusual to discover a mind fragment of a living person with the client. This leads to concern for the person who has lost or sent this fragment of consciousness. The attached mind fragment is returned to the body/mind space of the person with the help of true spirit guides. The Higher Self of the fragmented one is requested to assist in the reintegration and the ensuing process of reorientation.

It is important to do remote spirit releasement on the other person before the return of the fragment. There is a better fit without intrusive entities present, and the mind fragment is less likely to return to the client at a later time.

Marion

Marion was in her mid-thirties, a recovering alcoholic and drug addict. The first attached entity that spoke through her voice was her deceased boyfriend. He had died of cocaine overdose. His body had been found in a sauna.

As she went into an altered state, she had an image of the inside of the sauna, which she had never seen before. She was recalling the memories of his death. After his death, she had become a serious cocaine addict. She even knew where his supplier lived, though she never had met the man or been to his home. This had always puzzled her, and the session gave her the answers. The boyfriend was continuing his habit through her. He agreed to leave her and go into the Light.

One of the attached entities discovered in her first session was a fragment of her eighty-four-year-old aunt Dolly. A scan of past lives revealed that Marion had been Dolly's daughter in a previous life. Dolly loved Marion as one of her own children. With the assistance of her Higher Self and her spirit guides, the fragment of Dolly was sent back to integrate with her own consciousness. Marion immediately felt stronger and clearer-minded, and had more energy.

A few weeks later, Dolly fell and broke her hip. With trepidation, Marion visited her in the hospital. During the week following the visit, Marion felt increasingly tired and depressed. In her second session it was discovered that the fragment had returned.

Before sending the fragment back again, a remote spirit releasement was conducted on Dolly. There were several attached EBs with her, including a deceased boyfriend who had given Dolly some of his mother's china and silver after her death. His mother was also attached, still angry that her son had given her beautiful things to a woman he wasn't planning to marry. After they were released into the Light, the fragment was once again sent back, accompanied by her spirit guides. It did not return to Marion.

During a later visit to her aunt's hospital room, Marion played the tape of her first session for her cousins, Dolly's daughters. When they heard the conversation with the mind fragment of Dolly, they recognized their mother's voice mannerisms and inflections.

Joan and the Nanny

An entity can attach to, or be associated with, a subpersonality. The subpersonality can actually be holding on to the entity. The trauma that caused the split is still painfully active for the subpersonality and the strong need can be a magnet for the entity, even if it wants to be released.

Joan, a female client in her late forties, disclosed that she had not had a meaningful love relationship with another person and did not particularly miss the interaction. She suspected that an attached entity was at the root of this situation. Her father had died when she was about six years old, and she recalled standing beside his grave and looking down at the coffin. She knew her daddy was "in there," but did not understand why he would not return. At the time, she was wearing black patent leather shoes and a pinafore dress, and she wore her hair in long pigtails.

Direct questioning uncovered an attached entity almost immediately.

Dr. B.: "Is there someone else here with Joan?"

Client: "Yes."

The entity had been a nanny who loved children. In spirit she had felt drawn to the location of a cemetery where a little girl stood looking forlorn. The child was dressed in black patent leather shoes and a pinafore dress, and her hair was in long pigtails. The nanny came to comfort the child, and she had stayed. The child needed no one else; she had her nanny. The nanny was ready to leave but could not seem to lift off toward the Light. Guides from the Light were present. No other entities were attached to the nanny, and no unfinished business kept her attached; there was no apparent resistance on her part.

I addressed the entity.

Dr. B.: "Is there a part of this woman that is holding on to you?"

C.: "Yes, the little child standing beside the grave."

I directed Joan to visualize the scene at the graveside, to kneel down by the little girl in pigtails and hold out her arms to her. She described the child turning and running into her arms. Joan's arms wrapped around herself as she described the feeling of the child hugging her so hard. It felt wonderful.

I called softly to the nanny:

Dr. B.: "Can you go now?"

C.: "Yes."

The nanny moved into the Light as Joan continued hugging the little girl, her own subpersonality, her own inner child, her own self.

The present adult person is the only one who understands what the child went through; the pain, loss, anger, and frustration. The adult is the only one who still cares about the incident. The parents known by the child are now much older, if not deceased, and only see their child as the adult she has become. The child subpersonality is asked to trust her adult self, the one she became. The evidence proves that she survived the trauma that caused the split. She no longer needs to continue existence in the void of that suffering.

Nearly all clients discover these two conditions: their own soul fragmentation and entity attachment, some of which are soul fragments of people living and dead. The condition of fragmentation adds a new dimension to the process of spirit releasement therapy. Recovery of soul fragmentation is essential in past-life therapy and spirit releasement therapy.

– 5 –

Meeting the Dark Force Entities

There are two equal and opposite errors into which our race can fall about the devils. One is to disbelieve in their existence. The other is to believe, and to feel an excessive and unhealthy interest in them. They themselves are equally pleased by both errors and hail a materialist or a magician with the same delight.[1]

From ancient times to the present day, religious literature has depicted the polarity of light and dark either as a schism within God as Source, or as arising from different sources. Zoroastrianism, the religious philosophy founded in Persia (Iran) around the sixth century B.C., held the dualistic view that Ahura-Mazda, the being of Light, was all good and totally separate from Ahriman, the being of Darkness. This religious dualism was the first to posit an absolute principle of evil, a clearly defined Devil. A basic tenet of this philosophy was that the forces of good and evil constantly war over the soul of man.[2]

In our Western culture, even in churches, the existence of Lucifer, the Prince of Darkness with legions of demons in his command, is considered symbolic, metaphoric, even mythical. Whether the forces of darkness are a figment of imagination, a product of zealous prophets, a thoughtform creation of the collective unconscious, or something else unknown, speculations regarding good and evil will continue unabated.

In counseling practice there is little room for religious conjecture. If the client discovers such intrusive dark force entities (DFEs), we deal with them; we neither philosophize nor offer useless platitudes. For the purpose of counseling, the Devil or Satan (defined as Adversary) or Lucifer (defined as Light Bearer, the archangel cast from heaven for leading the revolt of the angels) is not categorized as a metaphor nor an actual being but as one aspect of the spiritual or nonphysical reality, a cultural construct that is meaningful in the therapeutic work with the client who describes these images. This is not a statement of belief or disbelief.

Whether it is imagination, archetype, collective hallucinations, mass hypnosis, a projection of the beliefs of the therapist, or something else again, dark forces seem to exist in some form and are capable of intruding on living individuals in this reality. DFEs seem to be present and actively involved in our personal and planetary evolution. Many open-minded therapists using the techniques of SRT are discovering the same types of entities interfering with clients.[3]

People seem to be susceptible to interference by DFEs in the normal course of living. Mental distortion caused by alcohol or drugs can cause vulnerability to such attachment. Sexual interaction with someone infested by DFEs allows the exchange of these entities. Feelings of intense anger, hatred, rage, and vengeance open the door for demonic infestation. Greed and desire for power and control over others—of men over women, corporate executives over their employees, rulers and kings over their subjects (and in some cases, neighboring countries), fanatical terrorists, politicians in positions of power—all create an invitation to DFEs.

A warrior going into battle will often pray to God for protection and strength. Such a call to God goes unanswered. God does not help one soldier kill another soldier. In desperation, the warrior may call on the forces of darkness for protection. The dark side quickly offers to "protect" this trained killer. The offer of invincibility is too much to resist, and in the heat of battle, the warrior says yes. And from that moment his soul is in bondage to the dark forces.

The offer of protection is meaningless, and like so many millions of other soldiers who have uselessly lost their lives, many warriors who have called on the dark forces for protection die in battle. However, the bargain with the dark side was made willingly, and the DFEs enforce such a pact. And because of the integrity of the divine spirit, the human soul honors the bargain.

The DFEs are hostile, arrogant, defiant, disruptive, and generally very unpleasant. They swear profusely, using obscenity and foul language but not profanity. They never utter holy names. The client may refuse to repeat verbatim what they say.

They interfere with any and every form of love. This includes self-esteem in the individual (even to the point of suicide), conjugal love for couples (this can lead to separation and divorce, even domestic violence and murder); and familial love and respect (disruption of family unity and loss of the healing potential of love in a family is a primary assignment and major accomplishment by the DFEs). They attempt to interfere with projects and institutions that can advance or improve the human condition.

DFEs understand only the energy of the lower three chakras: survival, fear, threat, lust, greed, power, antagonism, competition, control, bullying. This resembles the human ego at its worst. They can work alone, in small bands, or as part of larger dark networks.

The DFEs are ordered to cause as much pain and suffering, disruption and chaos, death and destruction as possible to as many humans as possible. They thrive on the pain of human suffering. They "feed" on the energy emanations of pain and anguish from human beings.

In an altered state session, an individual DFE can speak through the voice of the client and describe its function and its purpose for being with the client, identify its commander, and describe its reaction to the Light as the releasement procedure continues. The typical attitude and behavior allow quick identification, and the condition of DFE infestation is easily recognized.

A client's visual images of attached DFEs are described as an area of darkness, a black blob, sometimes with patches of red coloration or background. Black and red are the signal colors of the DFEs. Occasionally they resemble the typical red devil with horns and tail.

DFEs can appear to the client in many forms. Other than the black growling blob, they appear as snakes, spiders, scorpions, lizards, vultures, crows, ravens, bats, dogs, wolves, monsters, all with angry red eyes, frequently with hideous open mouths full of sharp teeth. They seem to be able to tap into the mind of the host, drawing on the fear-provoking images in the person's memory banks.

In the imagery they growl, snarl, or hiss, sometimes exhibiting a red tongue in addition to red eyes. Depending on the mental state and educational and religious background of the client, this can induce fear. This is the objective of the dark intruder.

When asked the name of their master they may call him Lucifer, Satan, Father, Lord, the Devil, the One, the Great One, the Eternal One, the Evil One, the Powerful One, the Dark One, the One who Knows, the Dark Angel, the Darkness, or something similar. They may refuse to state the name of their commander-in-chief or may deny any master other than themselves. Some are aware of God as their creator, but not as their master.

There is a command hierarchy of DFEs of many levels and strengths spread across the fabric of time, space, and dimension. All claim allegiance to the Lucifer energy. The DFEs are threatened with pain, punishment, and annihilation if they disobey their commanders or fail in an assignment. They believe without question and blindly obey the commands of their superiors. They are indoctrinated with three fundamental deceptions:

1. They have no Light at their center.
2. They can cease to exist.
3. The Light is harmful.

They are controlled by these three deceptions. This is the basis for the SRT techniques described in the next chapter.

They do not understand love, compassion, generosity, humor, loyalty, devotion, happiness, joy, or fulfillment. There is no reward for their services to their master. They believe they are allowed to exist and will not be punished as long as they obey orders. They continue to perform their duties because there is nothing else; it is what they do. Often they defend their actions that harm the client as "just doing my job."

It seems that the job is becoming tiresome for some DFEs. During a session, a DFE that first presents as blustery, defiant, and challenging might suddenly stop speaking. The client might take a big sigh. It is the DFE who is expressing in this way. Each nuance of body movement and posture, facial expression, and voice tone must be explored as if it were a communication from the entity.

After seeing this a few times in sessions, I had the idea to ask the following question, and I often receive the same answer. This was a great surprise when it began a few years ago. However, it seems these were not the first DFEs that wanted to be free of the darkness.[4]

Dr. B.: "Have you grown weary of this job? Are you tired of this mindless obedience to your masters?"

C.: "Yes."

Dr. B.: "Did you want to be discovered today? Did you want us to find you?"

C.: "Yes."

The DFEs can only admit this after the protective capsule of Light surrounds them. It protects them from being captured by the Reclaimer DFEs that will try to take them back to the dark realm and certain punishment. Being discovered, being captured by the Light, and speaking to us constitute failure. They do not want to go back to the punishment place for this failure.

This is just part of the body of information that has been developed from the descriptions given by thousands of people in the altered state of consciousness during private therapy sessions with many therapists, across the U.S. and in many other countries. Consistency of this information indicates the universal character of the phenomenon. It seems to be part of collective human consciousness.

The following is taken from the New Testament, Revelation 12:7–12.

> And now war broke out in Heaven, when Michael with his angels attacked the dragon [Lucifer]. The dragon fought back with his angels, [a third of the stars from the sky, a third of the Heavenly host, the angels who fell] but they were

defeated and driven out of Heaven. The great dragon, the primeval serpent, known as the devil or Satan, who deceived the world, was hurled down to the earth and his angels were hurled down with him. Then I heard a voice shout from Heaven, "Victory and power and empire for ever have been won by our God, and all authority for his Christ, now that the persecutor, who accused our brothers day and night before our God, has been brought down. They have triumphed over him by the blood of the Lamb and by the witness of their martyrdom, rejoice and all who live there; but for you, earth and sea, trouble is coming because the devil has gone down to you in a rage, knowing that his days are numbered."

And, continuing, in Rev. 12:17:

Then the dragon was enraged with the woman and went away to make war on the rest of her children, that is, all who obey God's commandments and bear witness for Jesus.

This rage of the dragon—Lucifer, Devil, or Satan, as he has come to be known—extends beyond Christians to include all of God's children, that is, all humans. He (the masculine pronoun seems to be universally used for this figure) commands his minions, his legions, the fallen angels of all ranks to do his bidding.[5]

Described in the Pauline epistles of the Bible, the angels (principalities and powers) were delegated by God to rule the world. The Devil is also associated with these principalities and powers in their role as rulers of the universe. Evidently, certain high dark beings are in charge of the activities of the dark forces in certain areas of the world. They can be assigned to offices and seats of power, such as king of _____, or president of _____. The power behind the Roman empire appeared to be the dragon-devil of the Apocalypse.[6]

The word "possession," as used in the New Testament, comes from a Greek word that more accurately translates as "demonized."[7] The unwilling, unwary victim of obsession by this entity is said to be demonized, and as such, subject to the full force of deliverance ministry and exorcism.

In these ministries, there is no differentiation made between lost and confused souls of deceased humans and the demonic spirits that are among the minions of Lucifer. However, Jesus implied more than one kind in response to his disciples question, "Why could we not cast it out?" He said, "This kind does not go out except by prayer and fasting." (Matthew 17:19–21) He said to them, "This kind can come out by nothing but prayer and fasting." (Mark 9:28–29)

In such an exorcism or deliverance service, the "unclean spirit" is cast out, condemned to continue its confused wandering in "outer darkness." If it is a thoughtform, mental aberration, or figment of imagination, then a process of "casting it out" might be meaningful to a suggestible person.

If a spirit is real, a conscious being, regardless of what type, something must be done with it. If not taken to a specific destination, it can return to the previous host, find another unsuspecting victim, or attach to the exorcist, as they sometimes threaten. Indeed, this has happened. It is like removing a nail from a flat tire and tossing it out into the street. The person who tossed it or anyone else may pick it up in their tire again.

The adversarial position of the Church fathers is without compassion for the possessing spirit, even though it is a God-created being. Regardless of any religious belief structure, the DFEs seem to exist. They conform to the historic description and classic behavior attributed to demons. They do not identify themselves as "demons," but as "darkness."

The word "demon" originated from an ancient Greek term, *daimon*, which referred to beings whose special powers placed them between people and the gods. The belief in evil spirits and their ability to influence the lives of humans dates from prehistoric times, and many early peoples believed that spirits occupied all elements of nature, a belief termed "animism." The Vedas, Hindu scriptures composed in India about 1000 B.C., describe a variety of evil beings who harm people. Christian ideas about demons originated from references to evil beings or so-called unclean spirits in the Bible. By the Middle Ages (fifth century to fifteenth century), Christian theology had developed an elaborate hierarchy of *angels*, who were associated with God, and *fallen angels*, or demons, who were led by Satan. Islam also developed a complex system of demons, called jinn.[8]

True demonic beings have never incarnated as humans. Because they have never been involved in human form and interaction, they do not bring human physical conditions, symptoms of illness, or emotional issues to the host as do the Earthbound (EB) souls of deceased humans.

An attached EB can behave like a DFE, yet the client will perceive the attached entity as human in form. Questioning the entity will reveal a DFE nested within the EB, influencing the attitude and behavior of the human soul. This may have been an unwilling victim of demonic attachment or the result of purposeful summoning of the dark forces leading to a pact with the devil. Appropriate release of the nested DFE will allow release of the attached Earthbound soul.

Past Lives and the DFEs

In a session, the client is guided in discovering the source, origin, or cause of any condition they seek to change or heal. The source of many human problems and conflicts often turns out to be an attached entity. When an entity is discovered and we suspect a DFE, several specific questions are directed at this intruder.

"What is your purpose here with [client's name]?"

The purpose is usually to stop, block, disrupt, destroy, "protect" from the Light, or in some way interfere with the person.

"How have you affected her life? Emotionally? Mentally? Physically?"

"Who sent you?"

They may name Lucifer as The Dark One or some other such description. This confirms the identification of a DFE attachment.

"How old was he/she when you joined in this life?"

More than any other time, the DFE enters at the age of three. Reasons for this have not been discovered.

"How many lifetimes, including this one, have you been with her/him like this?"

"Recall the first time. How did you connect with her/him in that time."

The connection may have been at a time of violence, such as sexual abuse, beating, burning at the stake. The person may have been accessible because of fear or intoxication, perhaps a warrior going into battle. The client usually recalls vividly the act of opening or inviting the DFEs. It is a dual regression of the client and the DFE.

In the late Middle Ages, opposition to suspected witchcraft became violent. During the so-called witch craze that rampaged through Europe from about 1450 to 1700, thousands of people, mostly women and usually innocent, were executed for diabolical witchcraft, and most of them were burned at the stake.

The alleged witch was often the healer, the herbalist, a gentle woman with psychic abilities who could communicate with the plants and animals. This unusual ability aroused suspicion in people, especially those who were dominated by the teachings of the Church. These women were often attacked by the very people whose children they had healed. Fear is a powerful force, and easily usable by the DFEs.

As the flames engulfed their bodies, many of these spiritually gifted woman, in excruciating pain, would angrily call out a curse against the townspeople who had betrayed them. The dark forces always energize such a curse, and the curse is carried out against the target person or persons. Also, the DFEs see this as permission to join the woman who uttered the curse in that moment of panic. They consider it an invitation, in effect, a pact.

Many clients have recalled existence on the planet hundreds of millennia ago. Even then, protohumans had a sense of the dark intruders. A number of clients have described these black things resembling pterodactyls, the flying dinosaur-type creature. These intruders seemed to descend from the sky in groups and simply enter individuals, inevitably in times of violence between individuals or clans. Anger would attract the DFEs, or perhaps the dark entities would enter and instigate the violence.

Such behavior is not new on our planet.

The Dark Force Networks

The DFEs can work alone, in small bands, or as part of larger networks. The dark force networks focus on specific groups or categories of people. Target groups assigned to the various dark networks include: families; women and men; gays and lesbians; physicians and healers, spiritual students and spiritual leaders; popular leaders of any kind; corporations and their officers; all ranks of the military; members and leaders of the Catholic Church, fundamentalist churches, and the born-again Christians; schoolchildren; political leaders; satanic cults; terrorists; religious zealots; enforcement personnel, drug users; and many others.

Dark force networks and their directors can be assigned to specific geographical locations, titles, offices, or ranks. It is not the person who holds the rank or title but the office itself that is the target. The dark influence passes to anyone unfortunate enough to hold the title or earn the rank.

The goal of releasement is to return as many DFEs as possible to the Light. And the clinical aim is to locate the directors of the dark networks plaguing the client. DFEs in such networks know no personal or geographical boundaries. Bringing the network directors and their dark networks to the Light has the potential of relieving much suffering in the world.

The Pact with the Devil

Many humans have made a "pact with the devil" in this lifetime or another, always for self-serving purposes. Occasionally the bargains are purposely struck; other times, the connection is inadvertent.

Once these contracts are established, DFEs are assigned to a person and they take control. When this human dies, the soul, burdened by the attached demonic entity, may remain Earthbound and continue to serve the darkness, usually by attaching to a living human and influencing their behavior. This is often the source of the nested dark entities discovered by clients in session.

Alternately, the assigned DFE can separate from the newly deceased human, who will then move into the Light and eventually reincarnate. The contract is immediately reimplemented when that soul returns to the Earth plane; the assigned DFE will reattach to the unsuspecting person. This human servant of the dark forces continues the work of the darkness through his/her own physical body, in bondage to, and totally controlled by, the dark forces.

The DFE distorts thinking, yet the unfortunate person actually believes he or she is in control of their own life. Without intervention such as direct or remote SRT, this relationship will continue unabated, the confused thinking well established, for many lifetimes.

In many instances the agreement is a conscious and deliberate act: summoning Satan for the express purpose of making a formal pact. These pacts guarantee some earthly gain—personal or political power, wealth, or sexual favors. The Dark One delights in proffering such pittance in return for the eternal soul of the bargainer.

Renunciation of the Darkness

Most clients who discover demonic interference can be cleared of the DFEs. Those that are released do not return. In subsequent sessions, however, dark attachments may again be discovered, as if the door had been left open. The DFEs will claim ownership or partnership with the person by right of prior invitation and agreement. DFEs do not understand reincarnation; they just know the pact was made, a contract for eternity.

Past-life regression back to the first experience of involvement with the darkness allows a client to take responsibility for past actions and behavior, sever the connection, and declare the renunciation of the darkness. The act of renunciation closes the door on the intrusive DFEs who claim ownership of a human being.

This works for a client who discovers a past-life event when they accepted the invitation or formed a pact with the darkness. It also works for an attached human entity who is besieged with nested DFEs. The client can declare the Renunciation of the Darkness for self and by proxy for family members and others who may also be affected by involvement with the dark forces. The process works for anyone who has committed this critical error.

When the client or entity realizes the terrible effects of the pact on themselves and their families over many lifetimes, they are eager to sever the connection and begin to undo the negative consequences. This offer comes like daybreak after a long, dark night.

"Would you like to break that false contract? Are you willing to declare the Renunciation of the Darkness and pronounce your separation from the dark forces?"

The answer is always affirmative.

"Listen to these words. Make them your own. Repeat them as your own."

"In the name of the Light, may God rebuke you, darkness."

The client repeats the sentence.

"I renounce all activities of the darkness."

The client repeats.

"In the name of the Light, may God rebuke you, darkness. I renounce all activities of the darkness. I revoke all contracts and agreements, pacts and oaths, rituals and initiations with and to and from the darkness."

The client repeats.

"Throughout eternity, for as long as my soul exists."

The client repeats.

"In the name of the Light, it is so."

The client repeats. After twenty or thirty seconds, I ask softly: "How does that feel?"

There is a deep sense of profound relief and peace, both for the attached entity and the client, following the Renunciation of the Darkness. The DFEs can then be released more readily from the client, and from the confused and misguided attached Earthbound soul, who is then guided to the Light.

The declaration of renunciation can be used with any client who recalls a lifetime when they interacted with the dark forces in any way, whether they were involved in sorcery, black magic, witchcraft, dark brotherhood or priesthood, or satanic activity of any kind.

We are not helpless victims of the dark forces. Through denial and ignorance[9] we humans have left ourselves vulnerable to these aggressive spiritual parasites. Not only can such invasion be prevented through awareness and self-protection, but the ones that are already with us can be safely and permanently released to their next step of evolution.

The DFEs have lost their way; they have forgotten what they are as extensions of the Creator Source. In their ignorance, they are stuck to the endless duty of producing chaos and disruption, following in blind obedience the edicts of their superiors in the dark command hierarchy.

− 6 −
Spirit Releasement Therapy and the Dark Force Entities

We wrestle not against flesh and blood, but against principalities, against powers, against the rulers of the darkness of this world, against spiritual wickedness in high places. (Ephesians 6:12)

The basis for Spirit Releasement Therapy is the certainty that all God-created beings contain the eternal, indestructible spark of Light. All else is illusory and transitory. The beginning of the game is outlined in Revelation with the act of choosing sides: Light or darkness. Every spark of God will return home, and eventually all will rejoin the Oneness. This includes Lucifer and his legions of demons, the "Forces of Darkness."

The process of spirit releasement of a DFE utilizes imagination, visual imagery, and invocation of spiritual beings of Light. This is not a religious exercise and does not require adherence to any religious belief. This is explained to the client before a session begins. Certain names will be used in the session, and specific beings may be called upon for help.

The spirits of Light who assist may be archetypal or imaginary. They may also be real conscious beings, existing in a nonphysical reality. These beings of Light seem to be universal and not associated with any organized religion. Spirit beings are eternal. Human beings have developed the rules and restrictions of organized religions based on misperceptions, misinterpretations, magical thinking, and personal beliefs, attempting to claim spirit beings as their exclusive property.

As the techniques of SRT were being developed, I looked for terms and definitions for details of the hypothetical model that was unfolding before my eyes and ears. I needed to learn small bits that form the whole in order to understand the bigger picture. I sought titles for various beings that would imply some characteristic or specific function. For example, Earthbound soul, a term that has been used for many decades, indicates a human soul that is bound or stuck in the Earth plane.

The word "demon" carries historical and religious connotations that produce fear in many people. I chose to use dark force entity (DFE), which indicates meaning without the superstitious overlay. Yes, these titles and definitions may be arbitrary, yet they are based on historical and contemporary literature on these subjects as well as the dynamics of an SRT session.

Warrior Angels of Light stand against the intruding DFEs, especially during an SRT session. Rescue Spirits of Light can be likened to policemen who arrest and immobilize the intruders, then take them to their appropriate place. For DFEs, the next step is the Light, though not the same place in the Light where the Earthbound souls (EBs) are taken.

The Cleanup Teams of Light gather the garbage and sludge left over from the DFE infestation and put the final polish of Light over the situation. The Cleanup Teams of Light can gather the dark thoughtforms, the dark clouds, the gray veils that cover the client.

Archangel Michael is a universal spiritual figure. I call on Archangel Michael and the Legions of Heaven to work with larger groups of DFEs, such as dark force networks, dark command hierarchies, sweeps of darkness that span lifetimes, and the DFEs that have infiltrated alien, extraterrestrial (ET) civilizations.

The DFEs seem to have specific functions with unsuspecting people. Descriptive titles were developed according to their function: blockers, stalkers, weights, trip-me-ups, watchers, imposers, reclaimers, enforcers, to name a few.

These SRT techniques were developed over the years through many encounters with the DFEs in counseling sessions with clients. It was a journey of trial and error. There were many errors, including the use of the classic exorcism rituals developed within the Catholic Church and procedures of deliverance ministry. Many graduates of our training courses utilize these same techniques in clinical practice to achieve freedom for the client and for the attached DFEs. It works!

As the questions continue in the session, the DFE will proudly declare it has not been human and would not want to be. There is no light where it comes from. Its function is to cause chaos and destruction for the client. This confirms the identification of the attached entity as a DFE.

The Warrior Angels of Light are called to form a bastion of Light around the work of the session. The Rescue Spirits of Light are called to bind the DFE in a capsule of Light, impenetrable and inescapable. As the capsule of Light squeezes tighter, the DFE begins to feel the pressure and its dark edges begin to fade.

Reluctant DFEs can be guided to recall the first memory, their first experience of being. Nearly always they can remember the Light of Creator Source. They were either dragged or enticed out, and promised power if they came out. For some reason they chose to leave the Light. They joined the forces of darkness and forgot about their Creator Source.

They were ordered to avoid the Light. They are kept in bondage to the darkness, forced into absolute obedience under threat of pain and punishment, and controlled by the three primary deceptions: there is no Light inside them; they can be destroyed; the Light is harmful.

In the clinical session, with the capsule of Light binding it, the DFE is led to discover the three deceptions in reverse order. The following is a typical interchange with a bound DFE speaking through the voice of the client.

Dr. B.: "What did your superiors tell you would happen to you if you approached the Light or if the Light came close to you?"

C.: "They said it would burn. They told me I would be destroyed."

Dr. B.: "The third deception is that the Light will harm you. Is it burning?"

C.: "Yes, it's burning."

This is often the immediate reaction because they believe it will burn.

Dr. B.: "Is it destroying you? Are you being destroyed?"

C.: "No."

Dr. B.: "Look again, is it burning?"

C.: "Well, no."

Dr. B.: "Did they lie to you?"

C.: "Yes."

Dr. B.: "The Light will not harm you in any way. Are you being destroyed?"

C.: "No."

Dr. B.: "Did they lie to you?"

C.: "Yes."

Dr. B.: "The second deception is that you can be destroyed, that you can cease to exist. In truth you are an eternal spirit being; you cannot be destroyed. What's happening to your edges as the capsule squeezes tighter?"

C.: "They're getting fuzzy, they're fading, they're turning gray—disappearing."

There is very little belligerence at this point. The dark entity's focus has been diverted from its assignment with the client to grave concern for its own survival. With a little assistance, it begins to understand that it has been deceived.

Dr. B.: "Turn and look deep inside yourself. Begin to focus deep inside. Tunnel to your center, to the very center of your being. What do you find?"

C.: "Nothing, it's just dark."

Dr. B.: "Keep looking. What did they tell you was inside you, at your center?"

C.: "There is nothing there except darkness, hate."

Dr. B.: "Keep looking. Through the darkness, through the layers of blackness. Keep looking, keep going, right into your center. What do you see there? Look carefully."

C.: "There is some light. Just a little spark."

Dr. B.: "They deceived you. They told you there was no light inside, at your center. That is the first deception. This Light is the spark of God consciousness at the center of your being, which gives you eternal life. Once you believe the first deception you will believe the second deception, that you can be destroyed. After that you will believe anything. They tell you the Light is harmful, that it will burn, and you must stay away from it. If you obey, you will never learn about the Light. How does it feel to know they deceived you from the beginning?"

C.: "I don't like it. I'm angry. They lied to me."

Dr. B.: "Would you continue to serve these masters who deceived you like this?"

C.: "No."

The Light inside has been described as a flicker, a spark, a little flame, a red coal, a pearl, a diamond, a crystal, a sun.

Dr. B.: "What happens to that little light as you continue to watch it?"

C.: "It's glowing brighter, it's getting bigger."

This always happens with this type of entity.

Dr. B.: "Move close to it. How does it feel? Does it burn?"

C.: "No, it doesn't burn. It feels warm."

Dr. B.: "Step into it. It is your Light, the center of your being. Step right into it. Stand tall in your own Light. How does that feel?"

Once the dark being has stepped into its own Light the darkness is gone, like throwing a light switch in a dark room.

C.: "It's warm. Peaceful."

Dr. B.: "How long since you have felt warm or peaceful?"

C.: "I don't remember."

Dr. B.: "Do you like it?"

C.: "Yes."

Dr. B.: "What has happened to your dark form, the darkness we first saw?"

C.: "It's gone."

Dr. B.: "Would you make a new choice? Will you choose for the Light?"

C.: "Yes."

Dr. B.: "Choose for the Light. Declare it! 'I choose the Light!'"

C.: "I choose the Light!"

Dr. B.: "We witness your declaration. The Universe recognizes your choice. And so it is."

This is the transformation of a demon, a dark force entity, and it generally follows this pattern. It is a straightforward therapeutic approach that can be learned and practiced by any open-minded therapist.

Dr. B.: "Rescue Spirits of Light, lift this one to its own appointed place in the Light. We send you to your own place in the Light. Farewell and Godspeed."

This is a releasement, or "exorcism," of a demon. Not from the adversarial position of a priest, not with rancor and animosity toward this foul thing, but from a compassionate stance of tough love for a God-created being who went astray. Long ago this spirit made a serious error of mind and chose the dark path. It has caused untold misery to countless beings. It has also suffered its own pain in the darkness. There is a great deal more involved in the process than this brief description would suggest, yet this is the final outcome in nearly every case.[1]

There has been criticism of this method of sending "demons" to the Light. Fear, which drives religious zeal, allows no possibility of redemption for those who rebelled against God. They believe the God Light, or the Heavenly place, will be contaminated by the intrusion of darkness. This view of God is limited and false.

These errant dark beings are transformed by discovering the truth of what they are. They drop their illusion of darkness before returning to the Light, and the place they are taken by the Rescue Spirits of Light is safe, both for them and the Light. They are the prodigal sons, and Lucifer, once a favorite of God, is the ultimate prodigal son.

Witnessing the transformation of a demon can be deeply moving. Some observers have wept during such a session. It feels like a holy moment. These are the dark companions, the devils described in religious literature, creatures scorned, despised, blamed for the misery of humankind, and greatly feared. Classical exorcism aims to cast them out, sending them to the outer darkness, without compassion or love.[2]

In his comedy routines, entertainer Flip Wilson often made the statement: "The devil made me do it." Frequently in our lectures, derisive comments are made, suggesting that spirit attachment is a convenient excuse for unacceptable behavior. The heckler is mistaken.

In twenty-two years of conducting nearly six thousand clinical sessions, I have never heard clients blame an entity for their undesirable personal behavior. People are relieved to finally understand the cause of their condition. They have always taken full responsibility. There has been no scapegoating.

The discovery of DFEs with so many clients was a startling and sobering experience for me. It certainly changed my perceptions of reality. Although the condition differs somewhat from descriptions in religious literature through the centuries, the condition exists and the effects are unmistakable.

Equally remarkable are the far-reaching effects of spirit releasement therapy. Not only is the dark one transformed and sent to its own appointed place in the Light, but individuals, couples, or families freed from this oppression have new opportunities in life. This is especially gratifying with children who are released from this influence.

The question arises about the reality of demons and demonic possession. In an orderly universe created by God, why would He allow such beings, and such a condition, to exist? Why is such chaos allowed? Some have speculated that this is His way of giving humans an incentive to strive for something better. The DFEs act like starting blocks for a runner, something to give the impetus for forward movement, something to push against in the journey home to the Light.

In the act of creation, individual sparks of consciousness are given the power of free will choice. This may be the greatest of His gifts. There must be some alternatives of great import upon which to exercise the power of free will, and it may be the choice between Light and darkness.

Of course, this is only a speculation growing out of extensive clinical work on this subject.

The Football Hero and Epilepsy

One major function of the DFEs is to undermine love in any form. Healthy self-love can be equated with self-esteem. Here's what happened to one teenager, a high school football hero.

Tommy was plagued with feelings of inadequacy. He suffered with low self-esteem. Though an excellent player with demonstrable skills on the football field, he rejected the claims made by others about his abilities. With guidance, he discovered an attached DFE. The dark entity had undermined his self-esteem and urged him to commit suicide. Tommy died in an auto accident, recklessly and purposely. He was held Earthbound by the DFE and he attached to Bennett, another student in the same school.

Tommy was discovered years later in a session with Bennett, now a thirty-seven-year-old man who had suffered complex epileptic seizures weekly for more than a dozen years, often while driving. His seizures began at age nine after he fell off a bicycle and hit his head on a cement curb. They continued for seven years, then ceased. The seizures began again when Bennett was in his mid-twenties, shortly after his first son was born.

Tommy joined Bennett because Bennett had bullied Tommy's little brother on the school yard. The motive was revenge. It was not difficult for the DFE to encourage revenge, as Tommy was already resentful toward Bennett for the treatment of his little brother.

The DFE was released. Some work was completed with Tommy in terms of the reality of his skill and success. He realized his mistaken perceptions and lamented his choice to commit suicide. He gratefully went into the Light.

Eight months after the releasement procedure, Bennett had experienced only three seizures. For him this was a miracle.

The Monk and the Viking

Organizations such as churches, the military, political structures, and corporations hold great power over people. Many people are eager to transfer responsibility outside themselves, giving away their power willingly to the authority of such organizations. DFEs have a field day with people in positions of power in such organizations. The old adage, "Absolute power corrupts absolutely," is directly applicable. Executives or officers, already buoyed with heady power, often succumb to excessive and unnecessary use of power with subordinates for their own ego aggrandizement. This is an open invitation for DFEs.

Institutions that have the potential for uplifting human consciousness, or advancing spiritual evolution in some way, are natural targets for the dark forces. One client recalled a lifetime as a monk in the eighth century. He had learned to read and write in the monastery, and later had taken an assignment in an Italian city to assist in establishing a university where many people could learn and grow. There was enormous potential for growth throughout the region.

The client described the project in glowing terms. Then the situation grew ominous. The "men from the north," were sweeping across Europe, killing and pillaging as they went. These were the Norsemen or Vikings, infamous for ravaging Europe during the eighth through tenth centuries.

They entered the city where the monk lived. He was helpless as he watched them approach. In a single blow, the Viking leader's sword severed the monk's head, and dreams of the university were destroyed.

I directed the spirit of the monk to look at the eyes of the Viking. The eyes were red, a clear sign of DFE influence. The networks of DFEs driving this siege of Europe were released. Questions were then directed to the Viking. His responses were repeated by the client. He had not been aware of the attached DFE; he simply knew his job was to rape, pillage, and kill. Secretly, he was worried about getting home alive, traveling back across the lands his band had ravaged. They had suffered casualties, and he questioned their strength to fight their way through to their waiting ships.

The Viking chief was used by the dark forces for the sole purpose of destroying any possibility of establishing the university. Killing the monk was the key to these nefarious efforts; the Vikings were expendable. In this case the darkness triumphed.

The Samurai and the Pact with the Darkness

Ryan was a willing participant in therapy. At thirty-eight, he was becoming painfully aware of inner turmoil, the relationship with his wife, who was several years his senior, and their family. They were in therapy as a family. In a fit of violent anger, he had put a fist through two doors and a wall. However, this was a personal session for him.

As he described the painful situation of his life, he had a growing awareness of physical sensation and the mounting emotion behind it.

C.: "Wait, something's wrong, something's wrong."

There were elements in Ryan's life that just did not seem to be right or fair. As he repeated the phrase, his stomach tightened. Suddenly he found himself in a past life, holding a dagger against his abdomen about to commit *seppuku*, the Japanese ritual suicide. It was the code of Bushido, the honorable way to take his own life. Yet something was very wrong. As he plunged the dagger into his gut and pulled it across his abdomen, he momentarily sensed the wrongness of this code that had led him to this act. In the next moment his second slashed downward with the sword in the prescribed manner of Bushido, and his head went rolling away.

As a spirit, Ryan surveyed the scene and once again felt the fierce loyalty to the Bushido code of honor. It was everything. It was more than sufficient reason to die.

As he moved back, exploring the life, details began to emerge. His father had been Shogun before being assassinated. His wife had been killed by the rival faction and a new Shogun had come to power. As son of the former Shogun, he was required to die and was given the choice to commit *seppuku* in keeping with Bushido.

Reviewing the death scene a second time, he had a different sense of the meaning of his life. Suddenly Bushido seemed nonsensical, somehow comical, yet enormously tragic. He realized that he had loved his wife and family and that indeed love was, in truth, the only important element of life. A major realization, but just a little late for this samurai.

Moving back into that lifetime again, he discovered that his wife was part of the rival family. They had grown to love each other, yet she was still a part of the betrayal. Her family could not trust her and had ordered her death. He died feeling rage at the betrayal, together with hatred and the desire for revenge. This set the stage for the ensuing events.

The samurai described his death scene without much emotion. He sensed two shadowy figures moving about in the distance. They came closer, their forms more distinct; each was the size of a man, yet amorphous and dark. They were spirit, nonphysical—definitely not human. They addressed his rage, offering him a chance for revenge.

They offered him reembodiment, not reincarnation, but through possession of the body of the new Shogun's counselor. The counselor was trusted and had open access to the Shogun. Certainly this would afford the opportunity for revenge, which the young man desired. In return they requested his soul, of which he had little knowledge or need. He instantly accepted the offer. This was his pact with the Devil—his descent into dark bondage by choice. The DFEs joined him.

Within two weeks the conditions were right for the counselor to be possessed. He felt a moment of confusion and fear, and the spirit of the young samurai just went in and took over. He adjusted quickly to the new situation, and perceived that the counselor and Shogun were walking and talking quietly in a garden setting. At first he thought they were alone; it would be a simple matter to draw his sword and kill the Shogun. With his hand on the sword, he suddenly became aware of the samurai guards following them. As he drew the sword with the intention of killing the hated Shogun, the guards reacted swiftly. The counselor—not the Shogun—looked, in Ryan's words, like sliced salami.

Here are classic elements of demonic intrusion. The samurai's hatred, rage, and desire for revenge were a magnet for the DFEs. They offered life, which is a deception, as it is not theirs to give. The divine spark of life within all beings is a gift only of Creator Source. The offer of possessing another is doubly intrusive: it is a violation of the free will of the host, and also a deviation from the spiritual path and a karmic burden for the possessing spirit. Blinded by rage, the newly deceased spirit of the samurai accepted the offer and thoughtlessly gave his soul in return. Revenge was not achieved. His foul desire was not fulfilled.

Such contracts are never honored. The DFEs rarely deliver what is promised, and this is the key to terminating the contract. The child of Light, the human, operates with perfect integrity and will fulfill the promise to the darkness, whatever the nature of the promise. Because DFEs never keep their part of the bargain, the contract can be declared null and void and the lost and confused human soul who struck that bargain with the devil is freed from dark bondage.

Ryan perceived this concept fully in the altered state, and was willing to reclaim personal dominion and his freedom. He listened to the words of the Renunciation of Darkness as I gave them, and he made the words his own as he pronounced the renunciation:

"In the name of the Light, may God rebuke you, darkness.

"I renounce all activities of the darkness.

"I revoke all contracts and agreements, pacts and oaths, rituals and initiations with and to and from the darkness.

"Throughout eternity, for as long as my soul exists.

"In the name of the Light, it is so.

"Amen."

From that moment Ryan had his life back.

Deliverance Ministry and Faulty Discernment

Dora was a plain woman of Mexican ancestry. At forty-five, she was unmarried, overweight, and disappointed with life. She knew she had an attached entity; she could hear its thoughts expressing the desire to be near and its feelings of ownership. In her quest for relief, she had tried various avenues of healing to free herself from this entity. Whenever it emerged during a healing session, she felt a dry, choking feeling in her throat.

A religious woman, she had sought counsel with her fundamentalist minister. He and two other ministers had attempted an exorcism by deliverance. As they shouted at this intruder and demanded that it leave, it responded with anger and violence. One of the ministers was slammed against a wall. This occurred while Dora was firmly seated in a chair. She had not touched him.

The three ministers were certain that this was a sign of the Devil. They terminated the deliverance service, telling Dora not to come back. This increased her fear immensely.

She brought a friend to the therapy session for support. Both were afraid of what might happen. As she talked, she recognized the onset of the dry, choking feeling in her throat and she was frightened.

The entity was an African youth who loved her. In an African lifetime, the two had been promised to each other in marriage. He was about sixteen or seventeen and was required to pass his initiation into manhood before he could join with her. Wading in a streambed near the territorial border of his tribe, he was gathering certain stones and other artifacts to be used at his initiation. Unknowingly, he wandered beyond the border into the province of a hostile neighboring tribe.

Suddenly three warriors surrounded and quickly subdued him. They buried him up to his neck in the desert sand. The hot desert wind blew sand in his face, his nose, and mouth. He drowned in dry sand. This was the source of the dry, choking feeling in Dora's throat.

In spirit he returned to his village. It was tradition that a place for the departed spirit be set at table. He joined the others; they could not see him and did not acknowledge his presence. His intended bride grieved and obviously ignored him. He wandered outside in the village. Spirits of deceased warriors stood guard around the settlement. They had remained Earthbound. Eventually he left the area, wandering aimlessly. He found Dora in the present lifetime when she was about the age of his bride-to-be in Africa centuries earlier. Dora was the reincarnation of his beloved.

The ministers had attempted to separate this young African warrior from his love without explanation or any communication between them. Certainly they did not understand that he loved her. This was no demon. The ministers not only made a bad situation worse, they frightened Dora out of their own ignorance and fear.

As the young warrior expressed his deep love for this woman, he called her by her African name. He told her of his disappointment at losing the chance for a life together in their village. They both cried tears of joy at the memory of their love and the grief over their loss. He agreed to leave her to live her present life. He loved her enough to say good-bye. She watched as he was led safely and deeply into the Light.

The Earthbound souls of the warriors guarding the village were released from their selfless duty. They were tired and very ready to go to the Light.

Dora and her friend were relieved to learn there was no demon. This was a love story, not demonic possession.

False Alarm

Ben was a single father, a good father. His two teenaged children lived with him in a house in a suburb of a large Midwestern city. He wanted to do a remote spirit releasement to dehaunt his two-story house. Some weeks earlier, he had awakened during the night and perceived two spirits at the foot of his bed. As he sat up, one ran out the bedroom door, the other scurried into his bathroom. His elderly uncle had died some months before and Ben wanted to make sure he had not remained Earthbound in this house.

Ben had clear imagery in the altered state of consciousness. His psychic ability was well developed and he was able to thoroughly explore his house. He recalled and described the outside of the building. Then he was directed to search each room on the ground floor. He could perceive nothing out of the ordinary. Going upstairs, he searched his bedroom and his bathroom—nothing. The other rooms were clear except for his daughter's bedroom.

Psychically going into his daughter's room, Ben described a large black form on the edge of the bed. Naturally, he was concerned. We began spirit releasement procedure for the dark being. Warrior Angels of Light were in place and the Rescue Spirits of Light were standing by. Light filled the place. As Ben moved closer to the black form, now encapsulated in light, it did not move nor make a sound. He looked for the eyes expecting to see red. They were a light smoky blue.

The therapist directed the blue-eyed being to step forward out of the black shape. It was a female, hesitant and timid. She spoke. Ben repeated her story. This was his aunt, the first wife of the uncle who had so recently passed on. She held an infant child in her arms. Some fifty years earlier, she and her husband had lived on a small farm near the present location of Ben's house. She described her last day in her own physical body.

Late in the afternoon, as she was making preparations for the evening meal, she attempted to light the kerosene lantern. It was made of glass. Carelessly she put it on the warm stove. In moments it shattered, splashing burning kerosene on her clothes, onto the baby in her arms, and all over her three-year-old daughter standing beside her. Screaming, they ran out of the house, flames engulfing their bodies and searing their lungs. Ben's uncle was walking toward the house from his fields. When he saw the flames and heard the cries, he began to run. It was too late. His wife and children died before he could reach them.

The dark shape Ben first saw on the bed was not a demonic entity. It was the woman's painful memory of her charred body, the thoughtform of her death trauma. She happily released that burden. When she was directed to look upward, she immediately perceived the Light. In the Light she saw her husband only recently deceased, and her three-year-old daughter who died with her in the fire. The child had gone to the Light at the time; she was safe. The woman took the hands of her beloved family. She and the spirit of her infant daughter were lifted homeward to the Light.

The DFEs and Tape Recorders

We always make audiocassette tapes of sessions for clients. People usually want to listen to their sessions later, when they are in their regular state of consciousness, and often share the tapes with friends.

Much of the memory of a session fades like a dream upon awakening. Odd things can happen with electronic devices. In some cases, the equipment simply won't record during a session. It may be fine before and afterward, even with the same cassette, but during the session—nothing. Medium-priced recording units costing hundreds of dollars have been used as well as small units from Radio Shack. No difference. Microphones go out, new batteries go dead, electric outlets malfunction.

Clients have called with tales of their faulty tapes. Some cassettes simply disappear. On others, there are blank spaces during the dark entity releasement. No other part of the tape is damaged, just that part. Weirder still, clients will call months later to report that the blank section is restored, and they can finally listen to their complete session.

– 7 –

CE-VI: Close Encounters of the Possession Kind

In March 1981, I began seeing clients in private regression therapy sessions. Many people discovered what seemed to be lifetimes in Europe, Rome, Greece, in Aztec, Mayan, and Incan civilizations, even fabled Atlantis. Only a few recalled life in the Pacific Basin or Asia. Some recalled experiences of living in caves, wearing animal skins, and warring with other clans, using sticks and stones. A few narratives included encounters with large, dinosaur-like beasts.

Several clients found themselves incarnated in the area of Central America, in positions of leadership, in teaching, in healing, and involved with the priesthood. They had come to Earth from some other place in our galaxy, or beyond, nearly always in nonphysical form, in order to assist the "primitive" humans, particularly in the area of spirituality. In most cases, the people eventually rebelled against these leaders and killed them. After the bloodshed, the people reverted to their superstitious ways, which included meaningless rituals and human sacrifice. These peoples leave only sparse traces of their civilizations.

Some clients described life on other planets before coming to Earth. Some recalled living elsewhere, then being born on Earth, then, after death, returning to incarnate on their homeworld, and later returning again to a new lifetime on Earth. Some came to Earth in order to help awaken the consciousness of the primitive denizens of this dense, heavy planet, the humans and protohumans, who were so intent on warring and killing each other.

During altered state sessions, images and impressions can be vivid, the experiences extraordinary. Some narratives we have heard in sessions would make great movie scripts. After a session, the impressions begin to fade, much like a dream disappears after we awaken, no matter how much we want to recall it later.

In our SRT basic training courses, demonstration sessions are conducted with course participants. Certainly, individuals benefit from these sessions directly, and observers are able to see the techniques applied in real situations. The demonstration sessions are audiotaped. The subject of the demonstration receives the tape.

A set of earphones is connected to the tape recorder so the sound volume and clarity can be checked from time to time. However, my attention is riveted on the client in a session.

Occasionally I hear static from the earphones, clearly audible even though the earphones are beside the tape recorder. It begins during the discovery phase of the session, and ends after the intruder is released. In these instances, the attached entity is identified as an otherworldly being, an ET. If the session continues with some other past-life issue or entity releasement, the tape will be clear.

When regression therapy techniques are used to uncover the source of the presenting problem, the client may recall some traumatic event earlier in this life or a past-life event, or may discover an attached entity causing the problem. The attached entities are most often EBs and DFEs, though nearly half our clients discover ETs.

Discovery of the Attached Extraterrestrial

One type of attached entity is nonhuman and nondemonic, usually a highly intelligent being claiming to be from "far away," only visiting here on a mission. This is not the spirit of a deceased ET, but an alien in its normal, nonphysical form. Most have never been human in their own physical bodies here on Earth.

Of the many types of aliens described and categorized by investigators of the UFO phenomenon, some ETs exist in quasi- or nonphysical form. The ETs involved in abductions of humans defy physical laws, moving through solid walls, and levitating to their hovering craft, defying gravity. Apparently, some of these are able to infiltrate the minds of humans. Usually, people are not aware of their presence. In clinical practice, these ETs seem to be the ones we discover and subsequently release.

The Light in their home location is always different in color from the golden-white light described in the near-death experience and the past-life death experience in the human realm. The ETs describe their light as green, blue, orange, lemon-silver, lavender, or some other color. Some have been adrift and wandering for a long time and don't know how to get back "home."

Normally, they are not hostile, aggressive, or threatening, but intrusive and secretive; they do not like to be disturbed in their work. When discovered, they will briefly communicate and openly discuss their purpose for being with the client.

It seems there may be many intelligent species in the universe. If the information that comes through the consciousness and voice of our clients is valid, many extraterrestrials are already here among our population. And many of them are interfering with humans in the same way that other discarnate entities disrupt the normal course of life. If these discoveries are representative, then nonphysical aliens have infiltrated the subconscious minds of a great many people.

Attached ETs may be lost, marooned, or retired here on the Earth.[1] Some ETs are here on scientific expeditions, much as human scientists explore the jungles, oceans, and remote places on this globe. Some claim to use the eyes and ears of humans, as they do not have the proper apparatus to perceive this reality. Many of them cannot interpret the band of the electromagnetic spectrum that is seen as color, nor can they interpret sound waves.

Extraterrestrials express various reasons for being here, but have no compunction about the invasion, or hesitation in the violation of one's free will. Basically, there is no concern for personal sovereignty.

Some ETs claim to operate under the spiritual principle of Universal Oneness. Since they are part of the One, and humans are also part of the One, they are not interfering with "another," only exploring the larger dimensions of the One Self. This is an abuse of spiritual principles in the pursuit of selfish goals.

Alien Scientists

Some attached ETs claim to be conducting experiments much as Earth scientists conduct animal experimentation. They have implanted physical and nonphysical probes and various devices into humans for the purpose of location, control, communication, monitoring, and gathering information. Shiny, metallic nodules found in various parts of the body have been reported.[2]

As our scientists probe and dissect animals to learn the secrets of life, so do extraterrestrial scientists experiment with humans. They can control aspects of emotion and behavior; in some cases, the anger and fear function is increased. Then the experimenters observe human behavior in personal interactions. Apparently, they can interfere with any part of the mind and body.

Amy and the ET Clamps

Amy, a client in her late thirties, was trying to discover the cause of her impaired hearing. In session she uncovered a subpersonality made up of mind fragments of several different ages. The attitude of this subpersonality was: "No one ever listens to me, and I'm not going to listen either." We had to talk very gently to get her to communicate further. A subpersonality can interfere with a person's emotions and behavior, and this seemed a likely possibility for producing some change in Amy's condition.

When she was about four years old, a neighbor enticed her into his home with the promise of cookies and milk. He put her on the kitchen table, removed her underwear, and proceeded to fondle and kiss her genitals. She did not have any idea what he was doing, and she did not resist. It did not hurt; it felt rather good. When she got home, she told her mother.

Her mother blamed and shamed her, and did not confront the

neighbor. Her mother simply would not listen to her, she just scolded. The girl felt her mother was rejecting her for doing something wrong, though she never explained what it was. Her image of the memory was of her mother pounding on her uterus. She felt dirty, contaminated.

As an adult, if a man chastises her about something or makes her feel rejected, she reacts like a petulant child, although she realizes she overreacts in such situations. Using these thoughts, and the feelings of contamination and dirtiness, I guided her to another lifetime.

"Are these feelings familiar to you?"

They were familiar. This was not a new sensation.

"Recall another time when you felt the same way. Recall another time and place when you felt like this."

The images began to form within a minute. A young woman in a prominent family, she was well known in her small town. One evening she was walking home; it was nearly dark and she knew it was not safe to be out so late. She was accosted by five young toughs, taken to a nearby barn, tied, and gang-raped. She was not found until morning.

She was taken to the local doctor, who openly showed disgust and barely touched her during the examination. She was deeply hurt and humiliated as other people avoided her. At home, her old black maid cried as she cleaned up the young girl, who had been a virgin. She never married. She could never scrub herself sufficiently to feel clean. She died feeling dirty and contaminated. This feeling was restimulated when her mother in this life scolded her for telling about the neighbor who molested her.

There were DFEs involved, inciting the young toughs to carry out the rape, and the dark, contaminating residue remained with her. The residue from that experience was cleared. The subpersonality in this life immediately felt okay, not dirty, and was not so hesitant to talk with us. This hearing problem involved a subpersonality, past-life trauma, and DFEs. Now something else emerged.

As the four-year-old subpersonality was finally willing to take her rightful places (since she was made up of several fragments), Amy described a double sliding door interfering with the hearing.

"Focus on the sliding door. If you could know the source of that, what would it be?"

She described a fleeting image of two metallic, mechanical claws or clamps on both sides of her head. Further probing revealed an alien experiment on the sense organs. The experimenters wanted to observe the effect on other sense organs, such as sight and touch, if the sense of hearing was reduced. This was the primary cause of the hearing loss. Amy's hearing improved following the session, but was not restored to normal levels.

The other influences contributed to the condition, but ETs were at the core of the problem. With just a little persuasion, the commander aboard the space station agreed to remove the devices from Amy, and cease all such experimentation on humans. He had not designed the experiments, he was just carrying out orders. We could discover no DFEs behind this project; the ETs claimed it was purely a science project.

Jenna and the ET/DFE Connection

Jenna discovered an ET group experimenting with her sexuality. The ET scientists would intensify her sex drive, rather like increasing the volume on a TV set, then observe her behavior and the reactions to her own behavior. She expressed dismay at her sexual appetite and her promiscuity. This condition had existed in her life since late adolescence. She had difficulty maintaining relationships, and this caused sadness and confusion.

We discovered and released a large dark force network involved in this particular experiment, affecting many people. The ETs were freed of the dark influence and gladly returned to their own homeworld.[3]

Human beings are so caught up in sexuality from childhood through adolescence and into adulthood that it is a fertile field for dark interference. This problem is compounded by social issues relating to sex such as marriage, monogamy, adultery, and promiscuity; religious taboos, imposed guilt, unwanted pregnancy and abortion, human possessiveness, and jealousy add to the problem.

A basic tenet of science is that the experimenter influences the experiment. The observer is part of the observed. Thus the results of any scientific research must take into consideration the influence of equipment used, drug involvement, expectations of the researcher, and any contrived conditions.

This knowledge is used in convincing the alien scientists to abandon their research projects with human subjects. They may not have recognized the "experimenter effect" in their scientific system. I question them on how much data they must collect before they will be finished with the client. Usually, they are not aware of an endpoint, they just continue experimentation, sometimes through several lifetimes with the same person. Obviously, the attached ET researchers are technicians without authority or "need-to-know."

When it is pointed out that the experimental data is invalid due to their presence, the attached ET technicians are clearly distressed. It is not something they had thought of, yet they immediately recognize the validity of the concept. The project is suddenly seen as useless, a meaningless expenditure of time, energy, and resources. They agree to leave, eager to end this fruitless effort.

Clients have discovered not only these attached ET technicians and their equipment, but also unattended probes and other devices in various parts of the anatomy. These probes are nonphysical in nature and connected in a way that allows transmission of information to the alien scientists. The probe, or connector, may also allow the ETs to control aspects of the physiology as well as mental and emotional functioning of the person.

In an altered state of consciousness, a client can visualize the probe leading to the ET laboratory. We direct the questions to the alien researcher. The surprised ET will answer through the voice of the client. This can be distressing and unbelievable to the client, but with assurance that this condition exists with many others and the alien control is only temporary, most clients allow the dialogue to continue.

The alien scientists claim to be on a nearby spacecraft with many such research teams surveying or gathering information. The focus shifts to the ET command hierarchy, beginning with those in charge of the spacecraft. We are seeking to connect with the commander-in-chief. The space commander, crew leader, or the science officer is summoned. He will respond. This always surprises me. Why do they bother to answer my questions?

Lines of communication are maintained between all members of this alien crew and their commanders. They may reveal that they are under orders and part of a fleet of crafts on similar missions around the Earth. Additionally, they can cross-connect with base headquarters on the homeworld. The client can repeat the words of the base commander. In the altered state, this kind of "channeling" through the voice of the client is easily accomplished.

An outside observer of such a session might judge this sort of interaction as bizarre. However, once you get beyond initial disbelief, the dialogue between humans in a therapy session and extraterrestrial aliens in another dimension who are studying humanity becomes a fascinating study of consciousness.

In some cases, the base commander will acknowledge the intrusion, agreeing to remove the technicians, the equipment, probes, communication devices, any implants, and whatever invasive mechanisms have been placed. If the implant cannot be removed without taking the client onto a spacecraft, the device can be disabled.

They often claim they did not realize that humans would either be aware of the intrusion or object to the work. They give the appearance of compassion and quickly cooperate with the request to disengage.

We always request that the technicians remove all equipment, devices, wiring, and any remnants of the experimentation and the residue of their presence. Eager to do this, they offer an apology for the interference, often a request for forgiveness, and a hearty "thank you" for the new awareness of their useless efforts. They are sent home with a firm farewell. The client can feel the lifting of the weight, aware of the absence, the space now open. It is a tremendous relief.

In other cases, the ship commandant or base commander may be evasive, deceitful, even defiant, refusing to remove the intrusive devices and alien technicians. He will reveal that there is a dark command hierarchy that controls his people and instigates the intrusive behavior that affects humans.

The DFEs will divulge the real purpose of the "research." When humans are distressed by the intrusions and their reactions, they release the emotional energy of anguish and fear. The DFEs claim to feed off this energy and collect it for use by their superiors in the dark hierarchy. This situation requires the spirit releasement procedures for DFEs and ETs.

Alien Colonists

Some alien groups are intent on expanding their reach and establishing colonial outposts on other planets. This is certainly not a new idea; colonialism has a long and painful history right here on Earth.

These invasive ETs make use of the "carbon-based units," the living bodies of the human inhabitants of Earth. For them it is convenient to infiltrate people's minds and establish some degree of control. In sum, they establish "squatter's rights." Not hostile, but quietly arrogant, they are certain of their superiority. They are here and they claim there is nothing we can do about it. They are mistaken.

The Wanderers

A few ETs have no connection with a nearby craft and claim to be wanderers, lost or left behind by their crew long ago. We call on the Rescue Spirits of Light from their universe, using the color of Light they have described. It works! The attached ETs recognize and describe the colorful beings who come to help them return home. As they leave, they are offered one last chance to speak their farewells to the host. It is usually an apology for the intrusion, the confusion caused, and a sincere "thank you" for the assistance in finding their way home.

Another Language

In a few cases, an ET has taken control of the consciousness to the point that the client's voice produced unintelligible sounds: some kind of language, with inflections, sound patterns, recognizable pauses and shifts for sentence structure or questions, yet gibberish to the human ear. For the process of SRT to work, meaningful conversation must take place.

Occasionally, the aliens do not leave. In one case, the client's family had actually grown fond of the being who was living in their daughter's body, even understanding some of the alien language. With such acceptance and permission, there was no way we could convince it to leave.

Releasing ETs

When other techniques fail to work, I appeal to their sense of history and conduct a brief past-life regression on an alien attached to the client.

"Recall, in the history of your own homeworld, a time of invasion by a superior species. Someone from another place. Consult your computer, your libraries, the memories of your wise ones. (I use anything I can think of at this point.) Recall another time when your peoples were taken over by someone else. What happened? Can you recall such a time?"

There is usually some hesitation; it stops them momentarily. The instruction "Recall" is a powerful command to the subconscious. And they remember such an invasion by dark force entities. Is it real? Am I inspired in those moments by some higher consciousness to ask for such memory? Perhaps it is all just imagination—mine and the client's? Whatever the inspirational source, it works.

They will recount the story of an ancient time when an invasion occurred. I continue to probe, asking what happened, how the people reacted to the unwanted takeover. They see the disruption of their way of life as the result of conquest.

"Now you know how we feel about your intrusion here. Compare your reactions and feelings to our own as you come here uninvited. Can you understand our resistance to your presence?"

They understand immediately, and accept our request that they depart. They cooperate fully with the release process.

The DFE invaders are released from their people. The ETs are grateful. They agree to separate from the client and to call on all others of their kind interfering with other humans. They agree to leave together.

When the DFE-controlled ETs are discovered, the difference

between them is clear. It seems the legions of dark angels under Lucifer's command were dispersed well beyond Earth.

These dark beings plague other species with the same intrusiveness, arrogance, and disregard for personal integrity as they do with humans. They cause as much disruption, chaos, confusion, and make the same promises of wealth, power, control, and domination over others. This predictability allows quick identification and efficiency in the release procedures.

– 8 –

Birth Regression

The most dangerous and traumatic event anyone can encounter and survive may be the experience of birth. Sigmund Freud suggested this, and he may have been correct. He saw the trauma of birth as the origin of all human anxieties and the root of later emotional problems. A basic tenet of Freudian theory is that reliving is relieving, and that bringing the unconscious material into the conscious mind will alleviate the anxiety. Freud claimed that the experience of birth is too deeply buried in the unconscious to be retrieved in therapy, especially since it happened in the preverbal stage of infant development.[1]

This claim, of course, has proven false. Birth regression has become a routine practice for many therapists willing to take a step beyond traditional limits. People in an altered state of consciousness can uncover early experiences and verbalize the feelings of those memories. The infant can speak through the voice of the adult. The birth experience, conception, and circumstances prior to conception can be recalled and accurately described. Family members have consistently verified details of such narratives.[2]

One middle-aged client was guided to recall his first experience of his birth mother in this life. He described a girl of sixteen standing by her hall locker in high school. Skipping forward, he saw her on the beach at Coney Island, New York, listening to music on a portable radio. She was about nineteen. She was twenty-one when he was born. As a spirit, he had followed her for several years before his conception and birth.

Many women have reported being aware of a presence for some months prior to conception and birth of a child. Somehow they know it is the soul of their child waiting to be born. Following the birth, the presence is no longer sensed, as presumably the soul of the newborn is no longer disembodied.

Birth can be dangerous. Not only because of the physical event itself, but from thoughtless medical treatment. An increasing number of health professionals recognize the long-term effects of the birth experience, and there have been improvements in the process. However, the potential psychological effects of pre- and perinatal events are largely ignored by the attending medical staff.

Many contemporary therapists use techniques of birth regression to help clients uncover the perceived traumatic experience surrounding birth and resolve the emotional and physical conditions that stem from that experience. Human behavior tends to reenact birth; it seems many people are fixated or stuck in the birth trauma.[3]

Some cases of dyslexia, migraine headaches, a low-functioning thyroid gland, spinal problems, chronic pain, and other physical conditions can be traced to physically traumatic moments during the birth process. Claustrophobia, inordinate fear of death, anorexia, aversion to being touched, discomfort with tight clothing around the neck, and other emotional conditions often indicate unresolved birth trauma. Many drug addicts seek to ease the pain of living by ingesting substances that will dull the senses. The source of this behavior can often be traced to the moment when the mother was given anesthesia during the pain of childbirth.

Chronic physical and emotional symptoms are the signals from the subconscious mind that something is not right in the system. The symptom continues to erupt until someone notices. It is the inner wisdom of the body/mind that is screaming out for help. Birth regression can be a key to healing this continuing trauma.

Focus on your breathing. How are you breathing right now? Shallow little breaths or deep intakes of air? Most people find themselves taking shallow breaths, as if afraid to breathe, or worse, prevented from breathing.

This discomfort can often be traced to the birth experience in this life. As the infant moves through the birth canal, the umbilical cord is squeezed, shutting off the supply of nutrients, especially oxygen. Once out of the canal, the mouth is cleared of fluids and the lungs begin to expand and fill. If the cord is cut too soon, there is a period when no oxygen is available. This feels like suffocation to the newborn.

Birth Regression and PLT

Following these feelings farther back, a client may discover a prior lifetime when death came by suffocation, hanging, or strangulation. Past-life therapy on that death experience will ease discomfort with tight things around the neck and inadequate breathing.

Author and well-known past-life therapist Morris Netherton suggests that the past-life patterns that plague a person throughout the present life are restimulated sometime during the prenatal period, or during the birth and perinatal experience. He contends that past-life therapy on any given issue is not complete until the issue is explored in the pre- and perinatal experience.[4]

Recall of a past-life situation can be triggered in the mind of the unborn or neonate by sound or odor, the position of the body during birth, the attitude of the mother, or the absence of mother's consciousness caused by anesthesia during labor. The stimulus may be a word or a phrase spoken, especially with strong emotion by the mother or father anytime during the pregnancy, or the attending physician or nurses during delivery.

The consciousness, or the soul, seems to enter at or near the first breath. However, part of the consciousness appears to be associated with the body from the moment of conception, receiving and recording all experience, including the thoughts and feelings of the mother. This information is unfiltered, unprocessed, and accepted without judgment or discrimination as if these thoughts and feelings were its own.

This information can have devastating effects on the mind of the person during childhood, adolescence, and adulthood. Yet, these distorted memories can be corrected through pre- and perinatal and birth regression.

There are many indications for the need of birth regression. A woman may describe trouble with menstrual periods, conflict about an imminent marriage, confusion surrounding pregnancy and indecision about having children, as well as the emotions associated with motherhood. Often a woman can incorporate her mother's fears regarding these areas during her own prenatal period. These attitudes can follow from one lifetime to another.

A person might describe not being able to "get going" in projects, education, relationships, or life in general. These people are often late to appointments. In a session, they might discover their mother had a difficult labor, and this can be confirmed by asking the mother or some close member of the family.

One woman felt she had been "held back" in life by her mother. She didn't return to finish college until after age forty, then went on to earn her doctorate. It was revealed that an attending nurse had held her mother's legs together to hold back the birth because the doctor was late in arriving at the hospital.

Adult relationship patterns are often established during the birth experience. One man described his love life as a series of brief affairs with full-breasted blondes. In the session, he discovered that he had been taken from his mother immediately after birth, which interfered with the mother-infant bonding. He was wrapped in a soft blanket, held and cared for by a big, loving, full-breasted blond nurse. She smelled good, felt good, and gave him nurturance and nourishment. His mother was distant, not able to care for him because she was recovering from the experience of giving birth to her son. Now in adulthood, he was still trying to find the big, full-breasted, blonde nurse.

As Freud suggested, the trauma of birth may be at the root of later emotional problems. Birth regression and exploration of connected past lifetimes can unravel such conflicts. Freud was not a very good hypnotist and abandoned the techniques. Had he been more skilled in the application of hypnotherapy, Freud might have discovered past-life memories. Psychoanalysis would have taken quite a different path.

Birth in the Dental Chair

This event occurred while I was still a practicing dentist, during the first treatment appointment with a new dental patient. The young woman stated that she had always feared the dentist; she was tense and anxious as she thought of the anesthesia injection soon to come. When I picked up the syringe, holding it out of her line of vision, she twisted around and looked at it with fear in her eyes. She gripped the arms of the dental chair so tightly, her knuckles turned white.

In a soothing professional voice, I offered to help her resolve that fear so her experience of dentistry would be more pleasant. She agreed. Who wouldn't? It would be easier for me as well. Neither of us could know that she was about to be "born" right there in my dental chair within a few minutes. I replaced the syringe on the tray, then placed my hand on her shoulder to reassure her as I pressed the control button to recline the chair a bit farther.

Only recently (then), I had began to study age regression therapy. The "affect bridge," "somatic bridge," and "linguistic bridge" techniques popped into mind. At that time I had actually learned only four things to say in a regression session.

1. "How are you feeling in your body, right now?"
2. "If those sensations had words, what would they be saying?"
3. "Say that again."
4. "What happens next?"

Why not give it a try, I thought to myself. I was eager to test my new knowledge.

Dr. B.: "I can appreciate your fear. How are you feeling in your body, right now?"

Client: "My heart is pounding, my chest is tight." She replied without hesitation.

Dr. B.: "If those sensations had words, what would they be saying?"

C.: "I can't get my breath. I just want to get out of here."

She grunted the words between clenched teeth.

Her face began to contort, her forehead creased, her eyes narrowed to slits.

Of course, there was no lack of air to breathe in my air-conditioned office, so I knew from my studies that this must be coming from another time and place. Keeping my voice calm, I continued.

Dr. B.: "Say that again."

C.: "I can't get my breath. I just want to get out of here."

Her voice was tense, her eyes darted back and forth. She gripped the arms of the chair.

Still feigning calm, I allowed some emotion into my voice to keep pace with her.

Dr. B.: "Say it again," I urged.

The technique was working just like they said it would. I was getting excited.

C.: "I can't get my breath. I just want to get out of here."

Obviously, she was in torment. I wondered where this was going; my little knowledge might be a dangerous thing, though we couldn't stop now. Do not panic, I told myself, though I felt we were both losing control.

Dr. B.: "Say it again."

Her voice hissed with emotion.

C.: "I can't get my breath. I just want to get out of here."

Her eyes closed; she continued to grip the armrests. Her body jerked from side to side in the chair.

Attempting to mask my uncertainty, I added a tone of compassionate excitement to my voice.

Dr. B.: "Where are you as you are feeling this? Let a scene come into your mind. Where are you? Let a memory come."

I sincerely hoped this would work, but I wasn't sure. This is the way they described it in the books and lectures.

C.: "I'm in the doctor's office. He wants to give me a shot. He's trying to grab me. I'm trying to get away from him. I feel like I can't get my breath. I just want to get out of here."

She spoke in the present tense; she was deep into the memory, experiencing it directly. Her words about wanting to get out of here now made sense. Who wants to get a shot, no matter what the target zone?

There is plenty of breathable air in the doctor's office too. So her complaint, "I can't get my breath," still didn't fit.

We needed more information.

Dr. B.: "How old are you?"

C.: "I'm six," she said in a little girl voice.

Her body rocked sideways in the chair.

Dr. B.: "Okay, let that scene fade, and repeat the words again, 'I can't get my breath.'"

C.: "I can't get my breath. I just want to get out of here."

There was anguish in her voice now.

Dr. B.: "Say it again."

My voice grew more excited. The excitement was real. Uncharted territory does that for me.

C.: "I can't get my breath. I just want to get out of here."

Dr. B.: "Again."

I didn't know what else to say, having exhausted my knowledge of regression therapy. My eagerness to help way exceeded my ability.

Silence. She was gripping the arms of the chair, she held her breath, her body still. Suddenly her back arched, lifting her torso off the chair, supported by her heels on the footrest, her head on the headrest, and her hands on the armrests, her face stiffly contorted, and she cried out—

C.: "I'm being born! I'm being born!"

She paused momentarily, then cried out again.

C.: "I'm being born, I can't get my breath and I just want to get out of here."

Dr. B.: "Say it again!"

I heard myself shout. I quickly sat down in my chair. I had stood bolt upright when she arched up out of the dental chair and shouted.

She repeated the words, but much of the emotion had ebbed. Now all her words made complete sense. She lowered herself into the reclining dental chair. She seemed calmer, more composed.

I looked around to see if any of my staff had heard us. I was positive they had heard, but this was beyond any practice guidelines for the dental office, and they wisely refrained from joining us.

Comfortable after a few minutes, breathing easily, she opened her eyes and looked at me.

C.: "What was that?"

She was more than a little surprised. Maybe even more surprised than I was.

Dr. B.: "What did it seem like to you?"

I was retreating behind my professional face and voice again, not really knowing what to tell her.

C.: "It seemed like I went through my birth."

She was not quite believing her own words. It seemed like that to me too, though I had never witnessed a live birth. And never wanted to. I wasn't ready to agree out loud.

Dr. B.: "How do you feel right now? How does your body feel right now?"

Simple question; safe ground.

C.: "My heart isn't pounding, I don't want to get out of here. I can breathe just fine."

I was suddenly aware that I was barely breathing. I took a breath. It felt just fine to me, too.

Dr. B.: "Good."

My heart rate was still high, but slowing. I can't begin to express just how relieved I was to hear her say what she'd just said. I wondered if this was the way obstetricians felt every time they delivered a baby. I was glad I had chosen dentistry as a profession.

At her appointment a few weeks later she felt no fear. She was delighted to report that she no longer had any fear of receiving medical treatment. She also had lost her fear of driving on the freeway. There were other areas of her life that no longer caused or reactivated fear for her. I was amazed and exhilarated at the success of the regression techniques, and I resolved to learn more.

The course of her treatment required a number of appointments scheduled over several months. Happily for both of us, the fear was gone. The burden of fear she brought from her birth experience years earlier had dissolved.

After this successful "birth," I used the regression techniques with other patients with surprisingly successful results. So much of the fear of pain in the dental chair is connected to memory of past pain, and the anticipation of future pain. Some patients recalled painful events in childhood and in past lives without uncovering birth memories, and still released the dental fears. Regression therapy and uncovering childhood traumas really worked. Certainly, part of Freud's theories were accurate.

– 9 –

Past-Life Therapy in Practice

The doctrine of metempsychosis [reincarnation] is, above all, neither absurd nor useless. It is no more surprising to be born twice than once; everything in nature is resurrection.[1]

What is past-life therapy? Does that mean reincarnation? Do I have to believe in reincarnation? Do I have to be hypnotized? These and so many other questions arise when people think about the possibilities of exploring our own past lives.

Reincarnation

Many contemporary and historical American, European, and Asian authors, philosophers, scientists, academicians, clergy, and others have expressed belief in some form of reincarnation or continuation and reembodiment of the human soul essence. This stems from personal experience and speculation since there is no physical evidence for the concept.[2]

Dr. Ian Stevenson, professor of psychiatry at the University of Virginia Medical School, has documented several thousand cases of children who recall verifiable details of former lifetimes. These cases come from several countries including India, Sri Lanka, and the United States.[3] Stevenson also describes cases of physical evidence such as birth defects, absence of fingers, and in one case, absence of one leg, which correspond with past-life memories of physical trauma.[4]

In theory, each individual spirit is a spark of God-consciousness. It is eternal and indestructible, created and extended from Creator Source, journeying and experiencing through everywhere and everywhen of infinity, with the destination and eventual goal of returning home. Self-realization includes recalling our source, our destination, and the truth of what we are.

During this journey, some individual spirits participate in the reincarnation cycle of Earth by forming and extending a human soul, which is the life force of the physical body. The soul is also called the human spirit, and the terms "soul" and "spirit" are often used interchangeably, though they are not the same thing. Spirit, in the context of this book, is the human spirit, unless otherwise described.

The Light is an esoteric term that suggests a primeval source of total intelligence, the totality, the Godhead. It is roughly comparable in meaning to Heaven (Christian), happy hunting ground (Native American), Nirvana, (Buddhist, Vedic), the Bardo, or intermediate state (Tibetan Buddhism).[5]

After conducting many hundreds of regression sessions, reading numerous books on reincarnation and the few books on past-life therapy available at that time, and learning from therapists who were doing past-life therapy, I developed a clinical model, a simplified map of the spiritual territory my clients were discovering and describing. I needed to have labels and consistent descriptions so I could follow the client's process as the subconscious mind pursued their unique path to healing.

Fear or anger over some present life situation can uncover a past-life trauma, which can lead to similar traumatic events in connecting lifetimes, to the spirit space where the details of karmic resolution are organized for the present life, to the birth experience in this lifetime. The alert therapist must be able to follow such a sequence without losing track of the client's journey, and with some awareness of where, when, and what they are describing.

For this reason I coined terms such as "Planning Stage," "Review Stage," "Lifescript," "Advisors," and "Counselors." These terms are capitalized to indicate their significance in the model, much like Union Station on the West Coast, Grand Central Station on the East Coast. Other therapists have discovered and described the general organization of the spiritual reality using similar terms.

In the Light there is a Planning Stage. Several Advisors or Counselors assist the soul in developing a Lifescript, a map of the coming journey, a lifetime on Earth. The primary goal of Earth incarnation is spiritual growth and evolution. The mundane elements of the Lifescript include gender, birth mother and father, geographical location of birth, siblings, station in life, degree of wealth or poverty, and the purpose of the life.[6]

Along the way there are learning opportunities such as illness and disease, choice of marriage partners, choice of education and life work. All are situations that will afford resolution of the unfinished business and unresolved conflicts of past times, and six or seven possible checkout points, that is, physical death. There is always something to be learned by everyone involved in any choice point.[7]

The soul comes into physical human form through the miracle of birth, beginning with the joining of egg and sperm. If all goes well, a human being is born, ostensibly with free will choice to pursue the Lifescript. Learning opportunities are subject to choice. Humans are not forced to participate; one can decline the opportunity. There will be different outcomes based on choices.

After death of the physical body, the soul lifts away from the Earth plane and into the Light, guided by the spirits of deceased loved ones or angelic beings. In this level of the Light, the soul of the newly deceased human is welcomed home. If need be, the soul can rest.

In the Review Stage, the Advisors assist the soul in an assessment of the life just completed.[8] Were spiritual lessons learned? Did the soul progress in spiritual evolution? Were past problems and conflicts resolved? What was completed, what was left undone? Was the

Lifescript followed, the life purpose fulfilled? Was there interference? Following the assessment, the soul prepares for the next incarnation in the Halls of Learning.

There is a great deal of activity in the Light between lives. It is not just a time of rest. We are reunited with our particular "hive," cluster, or group of souls. We seem to return to Earth with these others time after time.[9]

Finally there is the Planning Stage, in which the new Lifescript is formulated. It includes continuing opportunities for spiritual growth and evolution as well as plans for resolution of past problems and conflicts, based on the assessment in the Review Stage. Many human conflicts require several lifetimes for resolution and forgiveness. Forgiveness is the key to healing. The soul again moves into physical form through the birth process.

This is a brief description of human reincarnation, the cycle of birth, life, death, and rebirth. The transition into the Light doesn't always happen this way, as demonstrated by the condition of spirit interference and attachment. The progress of spiritual evolution is stopped by such interference.

Details of this cycle are accessible to people in altered states of consciousness. But is it all just imagination? Could these past-life memories be active imagination, psychodrama, or just made up? Is consciousness a dream? Is physical reality just an illusion, as many spiritual teachings suggest? Within this physical reality, we simply can't know the answer.

The concept of reincarnation is an integral part of 80 percent of the world's religious belief systems. Reincarnation and karma provide a way to balance cause and effect, resolve the unfinished business of the past, and allow the soul to grow spiritually. Self-responsibility and self-determination are empowering for the individual.

The process of reincarnation cannot be proven through the scientific method, yet the belief has been part of human thinking for millennia. Many people can recall what seems to be real and personal experience in different bodies in other lifetimes. Past-life therapy is based on the model of reincarnation and karma. However, belief in past lives or reincarnation is not necessary for past-life therapy to work. It is not required of either the client or the therapist.

At the Second Council of Constantinople in A.D. 553, the concepts of reincarnation and the preexistence of the soul were declared anathema within the Christian Church as it existed at the time.[10] However, the pope, Vigilius, was in prison, the Eastern bishops refused to attend, and the Council was considered by many to be invalid. Because of this, perhaps the edicts of the Council are nonbinding on Christians today. There are many references to reincarnation in the Bible, though some are obscure and open to interpretation.[11]

Karma is the process of balancing every thought, intention, and behavior. It involves cause and effect, reward and punishment, action and reaction. If a person does something harmful to another, there will be a balancing. The perpetrator will suffer in equal measure, either in the present life or a future lifetime. A person can also balance a karmic debt by performing a helpful act. Karmic balancing can spread across many lifetimes. The operation of karma cannot be separated from the process of reincarnation.

In the framework of reincarnation and karma, an individual can eventually balance the books of his lives, so to speak, and fulfill the Christian rules:

"As you sow, so shall you reap."

And the Golden Rule:

"Do unto others as you would have others do unto you."

These are clear expressions of karmic balancing.

In this view, an individual is absolutely responsible for his or her life and what happens along the way. Blame is false, as guilt is false, because a being cannot hurt another being. Certainly the body and ego can be damaged and bruised, a soul can be fragmented, but the eternal spirit being cannot be harmed.

Past-Life Recall

Exploration of past-life memories reveals at least four levels of meaning of past-life experience. Superficially, it is fun and interesting to explore one's past, to see oneself as a farmer, a warrior, a seafarer, an actress, a poor servant, a lord or lady of wealth, in various life dramas. It is rather like repertory theater, with members assuming different roles in many different plays. At this first level it is an excursion through time.

The second level is therapeutic. Clients recall traumatic events in other lifetimes that continue to cause problems in this life. Some physical conditions of illness are eased or eliminated, and emotional conflicts can be resolved through past-life therapy in fewer sessions than with conventional psychotherapy.

The third level is a direct experience of spiritual reality: a broad panorama spanning past, present, and in some cases future, yet beyond time, space, and physical form. The soul's path is a spiritual journey, with occasional forays into the physical reality as a human with a body. There is a deeper realization of purpose in life (lives), a clearer sense of the meaning of relationships and love, and the vastness of the human spirit.

The fourth level of the altered state exploration is a transpersonal experience of being. For some people, this is a life-changing moment in which there is a disidentification with the ego and the physical body. The whole personal melodrama of life becomes less significant. At this point, a person no longer feels separate and isolated, but an integral part of something larger, inherently connected, and related to everything in the universe.[12] There is a feeling of oneness with the Creator Source.

Vivid or recurring dreams, especially dreams of dying, may be past-life memories. The feeling of déjà vu, in which a person seems to be reliving some past episode, may be a glimpse of a past-life memory triggered by something in the present moment. This can be a sound, smell, taste, body position, emotional or physical interaction with another. Some people have had déjà vu experiences lasting from a few minutes to more than an hour.[13]

Sudden attraction to another or an immediate aversion, may be traced to an interaction in another lifetime. When we counsel couples, they often discover they were together in past lives. And not always as lovers!

Strong likes and dislikes in food, colors, countries, mountains, oceans, weather zones, and most anything else may stem from past lives. Phobias, allergies, birthmarks, technical and artistic skills, language facility, even physical impairments can often be traced to a previous existence.

With the knowledge and wisdom gained through past-life therapy and the power of forgiveness, the emotional residue of past times can be healed. A person then can live and love more fully in the present moment. Past-life therapy is a powerful, safe, swift, and direct approach to psychotherapy. The results are often immediate and lasting.

Past-Life Therapy

When past-life therapy is mentioned, many people reject the idea of looking into a past lifetime for problems. They claim to have enough troubles in the present. However, when they explore present issues and conflicts in therapy sessions, the problems nearly always result from painful events in earlier lifetimes.

In a therapy session we normally don't direct clients into a past life, but guide them to locate the source of the problems or unwanted conditions in the present time. Their inner mind uncovers the time, place, and circumstances that caused the present-life situation. As we seek the source of current problems, people uncover emotionally painful moments and traumatic events in this or other lifetimes.

Clients seldom find luxury, fame, or wealth in other lifetimes. People claiming to have been past-life personalities such as Cleopatra, Julius Caesar, Napoleon, Anne Boleyn, or other notable persons are reported in the supermarket tabloids, but this does not occur in past-life therapy sessions.

In the Planning Stage in the Light, we plan the circumstances of life before we enter the physical state. The Lifescript is held in the inner mind, but we tend to forget it when we enter physical life. Past-life therapy is effective in accessing the subconscious, uncovering memories of traumatic experience, resolving the unfinished personal business of the past, all of which can lead to forgiveness. The result is healing the scars of the soul. A person can devote more of life's energy to fulfilling the Lifescript.

Hypnosis is not necessary to uncover a past-life memory. Emotions and physical sensations one feels while relating the present life conflicts and the words or phrases used in expressing these feelings are used to guide a person to the source of the pain.

Emotions begin to intensify as the client describes a personal problem. Emotional turmoil is the doorway into the subconscious and the past-life memories or images associated with them. Affect is defined as feeling, emotion, or mood. The affect bridge or emotional link leads the client to an earlier, similar incident or traumatic event involving the same intense emotions.

"Soma" refers to the body. As the emotions intensify, heart and breathing rate accelerate, the client may feel a painful sensation somewhere in the body, perhaps the head, throat, chest, back, or belly. The somatic bridge involves physical sensations that connect the client to another incident involving the same physical sensation, usually in a prior lifetime, often a fatal wound. The pain is embedded in the soul consciousness as dangerous and life-threatening.

Metaphoric phrases such as: a pain in the neck; my aching back; I feel like I'm drowning; I feel paralyzed in my life; I can't breathe; I just can't seem to get moving; and other phrases may depict an actual event in the past. Repetition of the phrase will intensify the emotion, worsen the pain, and uncover the memory of the past-life traumatic event. This is the linguistic bridge.

The emotions, physical sensations, and descriptive phrases together form the bridge between *now* and *then*. These are the bridge inductions or links for uncovering past-life memories, and most people will recall past-life traumatic events when guided by a therapist trained in the techniques.

As the painful memory surfaces, the client may scream in fear, yell in anger, burst into sobs, retch, or become silent and still, as if hiding. They may clutch the chest as if suffering a heart attack, both hands may hold the head or the belly as the pain of a mortal wound wrenches cries from his contorted body.

This abreaction, that is, acting out through words and behavior, brings a catharsis (cleansing or purging) or release of repressed emotional energy associated with the original situation causing the conflict. This release also extends into the present life to relieve emotional tension and conflict. It seems to restore and refresh the spirit. This is the essence of healing.

Past-life therapy is based on a trauma model, that is, the client uncovers traumatic memories that cause problems and conflicts in the present life and acts out the past trauma. Abreaction and catharsis are integral to the process of past-life therapy.

Whether these are memories of actual or imagined events, metaphoric, symbolic, even archetypal images, the therapist works with the imagery and narrative and emotions *as if* they were real. They are real for the client, and the impact of these memories can seriously disrupt a person's life.

As in dreams and the déjà vu experience, a client struggling with a problem is already entangled in the past event, perceiving it, feeling it, reacting to it as if it were now. The signs and symptoms of the client's problems, both emotional and physical, are often reactions to the earlier trauma.

A past-life therapist assists the client in unraveling the misperceptions and misinterpretations, the false assumptions and judgments of past memories. The client is carefully guided to a clear understanding of the actual nature of the event, personal responsibility for the circumstances, the greater purpose served, and the spiritual learning inherent in the experience.

This experiential learning and understanding can bring immediate and permanent relief of present life conditions and problems. It seems people keep working on the same issue of past unfinished business until they get it right, even if it takes many lifetimes.

This is difficult for traditionally educated and trained therapists. The standard model of the mind stretches from birth to death. Many therapists still go along with Sigmund Freud, who contended the memories of a child before age five or six were irretrievable.

When a client in an altered state describes a scene from birth, pregnancy, or conception, a past-life memory, near-death or out-of-body experience, an abduction by aliens, or sexual abuse in cult rituals, there is often an immediate lack of acceptance by a traditional therapist, even denial that such a thing could be possible. This attitude of therapists eliminates the potential for emotional healing of the problem. The client is left with unresolved emotional pain and unrelenting physical manifestations.

Carolyn Myss, gifted medical clairvoyant and author, clearly describes the body/mind connection. Every thought travels through the biological system and activates a physiological response. Some are like depth charges, causing a reaction throughout the body. For example, fear causes an increase in heart rate, sweating, and tightness in the stomach. Loving thoughts can bring relaxation to the body. Some thoughts are unconscious, yet still cause reaction.[14]

Traumatic memories and damaged bodies represent more than scars from events of the present life; they are the scars of the soul as well, not just the mind or body. These scars on the soul are carried into subsequent lifetimes, causing mental, emotional, and physical conditions. The conditions will persist until the past-life trauma is discovered, resolved, forgiven, and healed.

The subconscious mind retains memory of everything ever experienced by the being. This includes the present, prior, and potential future lifetimes, and the nonphysical realms between incarnations. Additionally, the entire track of awareness back to and including the experience of separating from Creator Source is embedded in the soul memory.

If there is anything in a present traumatic situation that is similar to anything in an earlier traumatic event, the mind will associate with the earlier trauma and the body will react in the present time. Expanding on the notion of mind/body connection, it is clear the soul memories must also be included; mind/body/soul is the holistic model of dis-ease and healing.

Past-Life Therapy for Phobia

A phobia is an unfounded fear, a strong aversion to something with no apparent cause. Such an inexplicable reaction can often be traced to death in prior lives. A phobia of water may be described as a fear of deep water, rushing water, or muddy water. It may be pounding waves on a shore, water over the knees, water higher than chest level, or water in the face. Often these specific details will accurately depict the conditions surrounding an earlier death.

Gene

The number one phobia among people is fear of public speaking. One client described his moment of terror as he stood before a crowd. All eyes turned toward him. It wasn't the speech preparation, the size of the crowd, or even making a fool of himself. Simply, it was the feeling of their eyes on him.

In session, this feeling uncovered the memory of a lifetime when cowboys carried six-shooters. He had shot and killed a man and was summarily judged and sentenced to be hanged. As he mounted the scaffold, he did not feel fear. He had accepted the sentence. As a gunfighter, he had always known he would die of a bullet wound or by a rope around his neck. The noose was dropped over his head, and he looked out at the crowd of people who had gathered. Ghastly spectator sport; all the people were staring at him. The feeling of their eyes focused on him in that way was etched in his memory.

At that moment the trapdoor opened beneath his feet. He dropped to the end of the rope and died. The sea of eyes looking at him was his last memory and the source of the present fear. The last time everyone looked at him like that, he had died. Following our session, that fear ceased to bother him. This is a good example of how past-life trauma can affect the present, and how past-life therapy can uncover the cause and eliminate the problem.

Maureen

In a demonstration session during a training class, Maureen described her fear of snakes. A friend kept snakes in cages on his patio, and she could not go through the door onto his patio. She felt the fear as she talked about it. I used the affect bridge.

Dr. B.: "Recall a time recently when you felt that same fear of snakes."

Her eyes opened wide and her gaze dropped to the floor. She wasn't seeing the floor. This eye movement indicates the client is suddenly thrust into the emotional, and often visual, memory of the event.

C.: "Last week I started to watch a show on TV and there were snakes."

Maureen pulled her feet up off the floor as if there were snakes in the room. She had instantly gone into an altered state, and her mind believed she was in immediate peril. The subconscious mind does not differentiate between reality and imagination, past or present time.

Dr. B.: "Let those feelings take you right back. Locate the source of the feelings."

The answer came in a few seconds.

C.: "I'm outside a building and I'm real curious about what's inside. I'm a man. I'm going through the door."

It was dark inside this simple, church-like building. As his eyes grew accustomed to the darkened room, he saw a table at the front of the room. As he approached, he saw a huge snake on the table, the dark, beady eyes focused on him. He seemed transfixed by its eyes and continued to walk closer. As he stood by the table, unable to move, the snake coiled itself around him and began to tighten. He died of suffocation as this constrictor squeezed life out of him.

His "friends" had invited him to this place. They were cult members who practiced death rituals in this manner. He felt fearful, angry, and betrayed. The feeling of betrayal became stronger as he realized how they had lured him. This indicated that another lifetime memory was influencing this lifetime Maureen was experiencing. I guided her in locating the source of those feelings.

Dr. B.: "Let those feelings of betrayal carry you back further. Locate the source of the feelings of betrayal."

C.: "I'm being pulled backward, like I'm just whooshing backward."

Dr. B.: "Keep going, where does that whooshing take you?"

A moment later, Maureen burst out laughing.

C.: "I just fell on my butt. I'm a baby in diapers and I just fell over backward."

She was a baby girl. Her parents were going somewhere and left her with a nanny. Mother and Father did not come back. She didn't understand. Years went by and she never learned why they never returned to her. She felt unloved, abandoned, and hugely betrayed.

I advanced her to the time of her death, and she experienced leaving her body as a spirit. In spirit, there is no barrier to movement in time or space. Years and miles are meaningless. Perception of events, including thoughts and feelings of other people, is greatly expanded.

Dr. B.: "As spirit now, move back and watch your mother and father as they leave you that day. What do you perceive."

Spirits do not have eyes to "see" with, yet they perceive their surroundings in every direction.

C.: "They are leaving in a horse-drawn buggy. I wonder where they're going."

Dr. B.: "Keep watching. Follow them. What happens?"

C.: "Oh my God! They just went over the edge of the road. The buggy is crashing down into a canyon. They were never found."

Now she understood why her parents never returned. This new wisdom erased the feelings of being unloved, abandoned, and betrayed. She could forgive them for the pain she had blamed them for causing. The blame was false. It was this blaming that caused the pain, not anything her parents had done.

I moved her to the experience in the church. Feelings of betrayal were gone, and she was able to leave the scene of the death with ease. This regression uncovered two lifetimes that fed into her fear of snakes in her present life.

Several months later, Maureen reported that she could now walk right out onto her friend's patio where the snakes were kept in cages. She couldn't touch the cages yet, but her morbid fear of these reptiles was gone.

Deirdre and the Black Lady

Eighteen-year-old Deirdre wanted to explore through past-life therapy her love of reggae music, night clubs that catered to African-Americans, her relationship with her boyfriend, and her fear of crossing the street. She was deathly afraid of being run down by a car.

Her relationship was used as the entry point. As she thought of her boyfriend, her emotional response bridged her into a former lifetime. She described herself as an old black woman dying in bed. Her grandson was visiting her, providing comfort. This was the boyfriend. The woman died. Instead of going to the Light, she sat on a hill and waited for another body. This was the first indication of a possible entity attachment, not a past-life connection. The Earthbound soul of the woman attached to a series of people. The last person she attached to before Deirdre was an infant girl.

When the girl was six years old, she ran into a street between two parked cars. An oncoming car hit her at full speed, and the child died instantly. The attached EB emerged from the child's body, fearful and eager to move on.

Dr B.: "Wait a moment before you leave. Look back at the little body."

C.: "Oh, there's someone else coming out of the body too. Wow, she's walking toward a door over there. It's real bright in that doorway. Wow, that's interesting. I wanna see what that is. Oh-oh, the door just closed."

Too late to explore the bright doorway, the EB went off in a different direction. Deirdre was about twelve years of age when the entity joined her. She brought a memory of Deirdre's present boyfriend, her affinity for African-American people and their music. She also brought a fear of automobiles, which she had suddenly acquired when the person she was attached to was killed by a speeding car.

This phobia was not the result of any of Deirdre's past lives, or the death trauma of the entity, but the experience of a little girl who died with an attached entity. The entity acquired the fear through the death of the host body, and imposed it on Deirdre.

The entity was confused about her next step of spiritual evolution. Deirdre realized the truth of this situation halfway through the session. She had grown fond of the black lady without even knowing she was present. I explained the situation and the consequences of spirit attachment. Deirdre chose to release the Earthbound soul of the old woman. The two had a silent, internal conversation for some minutes and then Deirdre, in tears, signaled she was ready. The releasement procedures were completed quickly.

Past-Life Therapy for Dreams and Diabetes

Pete and Marian

Pete was a thirty-five-year-old TV producer. He suffered from diabetes and required a daily intake of twelve units of insulin by injection. This is not a high dosage but it is significant. Pete had lost vision in one eye, and was suffering impaired circulation in both legs, which could eventually lead to amputation. Pete's body was giving out and he was awash in futile anger.

His TV show used the interview format, and I had been invited on it to discuss past-life therapy. Marian, the hostess, had reluctantly volunteered to undergo a past-life session in preparation for the show. The best way an interviewer can formulate intelligent questions on the subject of past-life regression therapy is to experience a session.

The session was conducted in a small studio at the station. A crew brought in a TV camera and set up the bright lights necessary for filming. Pete was also present. Marian lay back on a two-seater couch, her head propped up on pillows. Not the most conducive setting for an altered state session, but she ignored the circumstances and we began.

Marian chose to explore a dream that had been recurring two or three times a week for years. In the dream, she felt herself floating above a small, old-fashioned town. She drifted along a brick road to the edge of town, and the dream would end. She would always awaken feeling sad. Not the best way to face life each day.

I asked Marian to recall and describe the dream. She related the short segment, and I urged her to continue and describe what she experienced next. Surprised that her "dream" continued, she saw that the brick road extended down to a small river. The scene ended there.

At my suggestion, she started to narrate the dream again. This time, I made a clinical assumption that the "dream" was an emotionally painful memory, perhaps from a past lifetime. At the end of her narrative, I directed Marian to locate a time when she was in her body in the town. She immediately recalled an event and described it. My assumption seemed to be valid. Although her response could also be the result of my direction, what followed was not the result of any suggestion.

She was engaged to be married. She was standing before the smoking ruins of the home of her fiancé and his parents, feeling desperate and confused. All had died in the fire. The town constable assumed she was guilty of setting the fire and attempted to take her into custody. She escaped and ran into the surrounding woods, where she remained undetected for several hours.

She heard noises in the brush nearby. Three "highwaymen," as she called them, discovered her, raped her, then slit her throat. She floated above the treetops, removed from her body and pain-free, yet deeply saddened by the death of her fiancé. She was lost in confusion.

At my suggestion, she moved back and observed the circumstances of the fire. She discovered that her fiancé had set the blaze, planning for his parents to die, counting on their meager wealth as his inheritance. To his horror, he had been trapped in the house, and died with them. She was terribly disappointed by his behavior and by her own poor judgment of his character. Her naive infatuation quickly vanished.

She drifted across her little town, over the brick road, across the flowing river, and began to rise toward an approaching Light. This new understanding lifted her confusion and eased her sadness. Marian came out of the altered state feeling unburdened. She was also feeling vulnerable, which is normal following a session. She was a bit embarrassed to realize the crew had witnessed her emotional experience.

We always recommend an hour or so of quiet time before driving or resuming work following an altered state session. As with being awakened after deep sleep, most people need a little time to return to normal mental alertness. With her schedule, Marian couldn't do this. She rushed to fix her makeup to be ready for airtime.

After observing Marian's session, Pete wanted to explore his diabetes through regression therapy. It was now 11 A.M., and the show was scheduled to begin at noon. I agreed to do the session, even though it would have to be brief.

He went right into the experience.

Dr. B.: "How do you feel about what's happening to your body?"

He began to feel the anger. His eyes closed as he vented his emotions and described his physical sensations. The affect bridge and somatic bridge inductions are quick and effective in such situations.

Dr. B.: "Good, let those feelings take you back to another time when you felt the same way. Locate the source of the feelings of anger. Recall the origin of those sensations in your body. Let those feelings take you right back."

He found himself as a Native American hunting with a bow and arrow. He was stalking a bear, and the big animal was in sight. He shot an arrow into the bear. Not a good idea, I thought to myself, and without even a tree to climb.

The bear turned, chased him, knocked him down, clawed at him, tore his body open, ripping apart intestines and internal organs, including the pancreas, the organ that malfunctions in the condition of diabetes.

As he lifted out of the physical body in his spirit body, I continued.

Dr. B.: "Look at your form now. How does it appear?"

C.: "It's all ripped open, it's all torn, it's wide open, it's ripped, it's torn." He was already rising toward the approaching Light.

We had fifteen minutes left before airtime. I directed Pete to visualize light coming into the damaged spirit body from the brightness above him, to funnel light into every space. This was a good moment to use suggestion and guided imagery.

The spirit body, also called the astral or ethereal body, carries the patterns for the future physical body including the seeds of illness.[15] When it is healed in the past through regression therapy, the physical condition in the present life may improve, or the symptoms of illness may cease. If the wound is fully healed at that point, there will be no possibility of that illness in future incarnations.

C.: "Yes, it's pouring in."

Dr. B.: "How does it feel?"

C.: "It's wonderful; it's warm."

Dr. B.: "Is it full yet?"

C.: "No."

Dr. B.: "Keep pouring it in."

Which he did for a good ten minutes. I checked my watch at least twice a minute. We were very close to airtime.

C.: "It's full." He said this in a very peaceful voice.

Dr. B.: "How does that feel?"

C.: "Wonderful!" A heartfelt reply.

The now peaceful soul of this Native American rose into the Light. The regression was complete. We had five minutes to spare, and Pete rushed to makeup. An assistant patted my forehead with a powder puff, and I was escorted into the studio.

When the show began, Marian offered a few words about hypnotherapy and regression therapy. She shared what she had just experienced. Still a bit groggy from the session, she was not her usual "cool" self when the show began. The audience loved it.

Pete didn't normally appear on the show. This day, however, he wanted to share his regression experience. He was profoundly aware that something had changed within his body. With awe in his voice he announced, "I'm going to have to get something to eat. My body is starting to produce insulin."

Three months later I was again invited to appear on the show. A member of the audience asked about regression therapy and dreams. Marian related her regression experience. She had not revisited the dream since her session. It was simply gone.

Pete reported that he only required one-fourth of the amount of insulin needed prior to his brief session. A year later, he was down to one-tenth of his former dosage. His physician had no explanation, yet he did not negate the results. He acknowledged that the mind is powerful, and that such things sometimes happen. Pete was delighted.

These questions arise: What about other damaged organs? Were other parts of Pete's body affected? I can only speculate that this condition of diabetes and its emotional and spiritual consequences were part of the present-life issues. In his session, Pete wanted to focus specifically on his diabetes. That is what emerged, and there was at least a partial healing.

Past-Life Therapy and Forgiveness

Ours is a culture of competition, with such slogans as may the best man win, looking out for number one (myself), winning by intimidation, might makes right, lawsuits, loser takes the hind quarter. In such a climate, there are many victims: losers in the stock market, sexual victims, discrimination victims, violence victims.

When we explore the victim role, for example, in a case of sexual abuse, we examine the emotional residue such as anger at the perpetrator, fear of being victimized again, sadness over the betrayal, guilt about pleasure derived in the sexual act. There is also mental residue: judgments regarding self-worth and self-esteem, decisions such as not trusting men; and there is physical residue, including damage to sexual organs, scarring, inability to conceive children, disfigurement from torture or beating. Any or all this residue may remain with the victim through lifetimes.

There seem to be several mechanisms by which such abuse is planned and drawn into present-life experience. The ones with the most impact are balancing karma and bestowing forgiveness.

The old maxim, "An eye for an eye, and a tooth for a tooth," is a popular metaphor for the concept of karma.[16] In this way, a past-life misdeed of any degree will be balanced in a future-life event. Pain suffered must be in equal measure to pain inflicted. Simple, basic, brutal. And superficial.

As a client describes the abuse situation in this life, associated emotions and physical sensations may emerge. The emotional and bodily memories are fresh even if the abuse happened years before. The bridge inductions are effective.

Dr. B.: "Recall another time when you felt the same way. Let those feelings [emotional and physical] carry you right back to another time, another place when you felt the same way."

This may evoke early life memories from infancy when some similar event took place, even a minor intrusion such as cleaning the labia with a cotton swab. The client is urged to describe any feelings, words, or images that surface.

Dr. B.: "Recall another time when you felt those same feelings, another time, another place. What comes?"

This often bridges the client into another lifetime at the moment they were being abused in a similar or more brutal way. Men have sexually violated women for as long as there have been men and women. Has it slowed down in present times? Probably not. Let's take a closer look at the spiritual framework.

The client can uncover lifetime after lifetime when the abuse was echoed again and again. Anger and fear increased, extending to other aspects of life. All that is needed in therapy are two past-life events that mirror the abuse in this life. Then the client is guided to look for the source, the origin, the cause of the victimization.

After violent events from two lifetimes, the pattern of abuse is clear. The core issue is victimhood. The next suggestion will bring a memory that will unlock a chain of events, clarify the present situation, and allow for release of the mental, emotional, and physical residue in the present lifetime. Most important, it will open the way for forgiveness: the key to healing.

Dr. B.: "Locate the karmic event, the connecting event, the event which set the forces in motion that led to the sexual violation. Locate the other side of the coin. Trust what comes."

After a pause, clients will begin to smile. Almost without exception, the memory that comes is one in which they were the victimizer or torturer—usually male—in a position of power, sexually torturing another, or perhaps many others. The process is that direct and immediate. They see that the balancing has occurred, or has been occurring, lifetime after lifetime.

With a spirit being of perfect integrity, such abuse is seen as a debit on the karmic ledger. In the Planning Stage before a lifetime, an event is set up that will lead to balancing that ledger. Often the victim in the former lifetime will volunteer to be the perpetrator in the coming lifetime so the balancing can be complete.

However, once in the lifetime, such plans are forgotten, and the ego and our violent emotions cloud the deep memories and interfere with the balancing. And the cycle continues.

Dual Regression

Past-life therapy is important in couples counseling. A dual regression can be a fascinating experience for two people. Usually the two people locate the same lifetime, but not always. In this case, they found the same experience immediately.

Gail and Stan

Gail and Stan seemed very much in love. Stan had experienced a past-life regression several months before he met Gail. He recalled a life in a small town in Idaho in the 1800s. The session was meaningful to him. In that life, he was married, feeling a deeply loving connection with his wife. Though she died at a fairly young age, he raised their children and attained some political prominence in the town. It was a good life.

When the two met in this life, they felt a strong mutual attraction.

In an intimate moment, Stan described to her his past-life regression in Idaho. He looked at her and was stunned, recognizing Gail as his beloved wife in the earlier lifetime. They wanted to be regressed together.

A garden meditation took them into an altered state. They visualized the colors of the flowers, felt the strength of the trees, and passed out a gate at the end of the garden. They were directed to a time when they had known each other. Gail was the first to speak.

Gail: "There is a wavy motion. We're moving."

Stan: "You're scared."

G.: "I'm not scared. We're on a sailing ship. We're going somewhere."

Dr. B.: "Where are you coming from?"

A gentle probing question often focuses the recall into more specific details.

G.: "England. We're going to the New World for some reason. Where is our luggage? Where are the children? I am scared."

S.: "We've been accused of doing something. We're going to the prison colonies. The children were left with your sister in London."

Their names were Henry and Angela. They were in love. They had been accused of some minor crime and were being exiled to the prison colonies in the New World that would eventually become America. He made a promise to her that he would take her back to see the children. It was a promise he never kept.

A few months later she became ill. Henry reminded her of his promise to reunite her with their children. She could not hold on. Angela cried with deep sobs, knowing she would never see them again. As she died quietly, he was also sobbing, heartbroken. Silently he vowed to her that they would be together again.

After a pause, we continued:

Dr. B.: "Are there any promises you make to each other before you leave the body?"

G.: "I'll always love you, Henry."

S.: "I'll always love you. I can never give you children."

Dr. B.: "Skip to the very moment you leave the body, Angela. What happens?"

141

G.: "I'm out of the body, I'm up above it."

Dr. B.: "How does it feel, floating above your body?"

G.: "I'm free."

Stan was still crying. Gail's voice was peaceful and soft. She was concerned about Henry. He was grieving and crying. She could not help him, and she began to cry.

G.: "I feel so bad that he is grieving. I left him down there all alone. I wish he could be here. It's so much better here."

Dr. B.: "He can't know that from where he is now. And there is nothing you can do about it. What do you do next, Angela?"

G.: "Floating, higher and higher, becoming smaller, like a point. It was like one little problem out of so many all around. There were problems all around the world. So many."

Dr. B.: "Look around. Can you see anyone else? Can you see your children?"

Gail burst out crying and laughing simultaneously. She recognized her children in spirit. They had died in England and Henry and Angela, across the Atlantic, never knew. Now she was with them and feeling great joy in the reunion.

This did not disturb Stan's experience. He continued with his narrative.

Several years later, Henry returned to London to find their two children. He was wary and careful; he was still considered a criminal in London. He went to the sister's house only to learn that the children, Michael and Christina, had died of illness. He felt he had let Angela down again.

Stan jerked in the chair.

Dr. B.: "What happened, what just happened?"

S.: "It's finished. I'm ready to go. It's over."

In his depressed state he wandered the back streets of London. A group of young toughs attacked Henry, beating him unmercifully.

S.: "Oooh! Ow! That did it."

Dr. B.: "What happened?"

S.: "Someone clobbered me right on the head."

Dr. B.: "What happens next?"

S.: "My body relaxes. They got the wrong man. But it doesn't matter."

Dr. B.: "Remember your thoughts about being finished, ready to go? For your purposes, did they get the wrong man?"

S.: (laughing) "No. I don't think so. I'm done. I'm up out of my body."

Dr. B.: (more softly, to Gail) "Dear one, as this is happening to him, can you see him from where you are?"

G.: "Oh yeah." (joyful laughter)

Dr. B.: "He doesn't see you yet, does he?"

G.: "No."

Dr. B.: (more firmly, to Stan) "What happens to you next?"

S.: "I hang around watching them beating my body. It is absurd. I'm just loving them. It's time for me to rest now."

Dr. B.: "Keep looking around. What do you experience?"

S.: "Well, there are the heavens, the stars. I never pictured anything like this. There is a lot of swirling. A lot of stars rushing by, and they got thicker and thicker. There's a lot of white. A lot of white light all around. And it's like I see Angela's eyes looking through. (laughter) I know she doesn't need to have a form, but I still need her to have a form."

Dr. B.: "Yes, the eyes are the windows of the soul. It's how we recognize each other. She would give you that form so you could recognize her. Later you will recognize her by her vibration."

S.: "Yeah."

Dr. B.: "How is it now, being together in that space?"

G.: "Ecstasy."

S.: (laughing with her) "Wow. It's like there is no separation. Wispy . . ."

Both their voices trailed off, their faces displayed peaceful joy.

Dr. B.: "Exactly so. There is no separation in the inner being. There is only *one*, only the blending and connecting of consciousness. In human form, this is what we seek without knowing what it is that we long for."

S.: "It's like one long orgasm. There is no beginning, no ending."

They laughed together.

Dr. B.: "This is true communication, to blend in spirit. It is what we know deep within ourselves. It is what we remember. And it is the ego that holds to the illusion of separation. In spirit we are all one. This is the experience."

They enjoyed the bliss for a few minutes and were ready to move further. They explored the life together in Idaho that Stan had previously recalled. In the third lifetime, Gail found herself as a Brazilian attorney, single and very active in amorous pursuits. Stan experienced being an older married Chinese peasant woman. They were surprised by this switch. They never connected in that lifetime.

A few months after this dual regression, Gail and Stan dissolved their relationship, without rancor, blame, guilt, or negative feelings. They parted in peace and love. They were not soul mates but they did have that lifetime of pain and regret to heal and forgive.

Group Regression

Groups of people can be guided in past-life exploration, the first level of past-life recall. Most individuals discover prior life experiences, couples often find the same lifetime. Within a group of people attending a seminar or training course, two or more will usually recognize several others in the group. The similarity of interest will draw the same people together again, perhaps for many lifetimes.

In our two-day past-life regression seminars, we conduct seven regressions. Participants are guided to locate the past-life source of certain emotions in their present lives: anger, fear, sadness, guilt, and feelings of abandonment. They are directed to explore a significant relationship. They are also guided to learn their purpose in life.

The instruction for the regression on one's purpose in life is explicit: Locate the moment when you first chose to come to the planet Earth.

The results are surprising. Over the last two decades, between 60 percent and 70 percent of participants recall coming into Earth existence from another planet or dimension. The purpose is to bring healing, love, and light to people here, and to help them overcome the heaviness and darkness that pervade this planet. Many humans have forgotten their origin, their Source, their spark of God-Light within. Other seminar leaders conducting group regressions regarding purpose in life often find similar results.

Past-Life Recall as an Extraterrestrial

The suggestions "recall" and "locate" are powerful commands to the subconscious. If those levels of "mind" called subconscious and unconscious actually carry soul memories of other lives, the space between lives, and existence on other worlds, then these "memories" are available through regression therapy. If these narratives are imagination, my mind boggles at the variegated richness of the human imagination in all its dimensions.

As one woman recalled her life on another world, she described it as "returning home for further instructions" before continuing in a long series of Earth lifetimes. She was a teacher and healer; she believed it was her job to bring that energy to Earth.

A highly intelligent young man, seriously depressed and feeling lost in life, recalled his origins on another planet. He was part of a group of students of higher learning there, and his trip to Earth for an incarnation was nothing more than a field trip for this group. He had lost contact with them and felt alone in his mission. As he touched into the consciousness of his group, he learned that many of them had also forgotten their mission, and several had committed suicide. With this knowledge, his depression eased and he regained his enthusiasm for following the spiritual path of learning; and I suspect he will go on to fulfill his assignment here on this field trip to Earth.

One type of alien being reported often in recent years has become identified as the "Nordic" type. Blond, blue-eyed, kindly and helpful. Apparently these types have been coming to Earth for millennia.

Most of our clients living in the United States find past lives in Central and South America, Western European countries, the Holy Land, Egypt, and before that, Atlantis. Soul migration seems to be mostly from East to West. Many narratives indicate that the exodus from Atlantis in its last days took people eastward to Africa and the European continent, and westward to the South American lands. From those areas they migrated northward, both physically and by reincarnation.

Ted

Ted attended our basic SRT training course. As a hypnotherapist, he wanted to expand his knowledge and skills. He volunteered as a demonstration subject. Though not uncommon, the tale that emerged was disturbing to Ted.

He discovered a small group of attached ETs that had been in place for years. That's not unusual. Its stated purpose was to gather data on humans in normal life circumstances. Again, that's a common situation. What came next was unusual, though we have heard it in other sessions. I directed Ted to locate the origin of this ET connection. He was very surprised at what his own subconscious mind and the ET leader disclosed.

Prior to the present lifetime, Ted was an associate of the attached ETs. They knew each other as fellow citizens on another planet. Ted himself was an ET. His past lives were on another planet. This knowledge was hard for him to accept, yet there it was, coming from his own memory banks.

As part of a "scientific" team on the other planet, Ted agreed to come into the Earth cycle as a research subject. As a human being, he would be a living laboratory for his teammates to study without the hostility or resistance that a native Earth inhabitant might exhibit.

These former coworkers followed him to Earth, moved into his body when Ted was very young, and had set up their equipment. Whatever the effects, he was used to them since they had been present nearly all his life.

Ted chose to release the ETs, get rid of the equipment, the communication and control devices that had been implanted. He disliked what he had discovered about his own past, and he chose a different course. He abandoned the alien project and chose human life. The ETs honored his choice; they knew his free will choice was one of the possible outcomes of such experimentation if Ted discovered them. They agreed to return to their own home-world.

Future Life Progression

Future-life experience is nearly as accessible as past lives. Occasionally a client will describe a traumatic event in a future life as the source of a present-life problem.[17] A client can find resolution of present-life problems with the future-lives progression as easily as with past lives regression.

Lifetimes do not always line up like a string of pearls, though clients often perceive their past lives in sequential order. One client in a deep altered state described her many lifetimes as "bubbles of time" floating in space and she could choose to go into any of them. She knew if she resolved her conflicts and completed her unfinished business in one, several other potential lives would no longer be necessary and they would disappear from the scene.

In the nonphysical realm, time is not a sequence of events, as it seems to be in our physical space-time continuum. Quantum physicists tell us time does not exist as we perceive and measure it. Mystics contend that time is nonexistent; all events occur simultaneously.

The past-life therapist works within this paradigm that contains time and no-time without attempting to explain the unknown and unknowable. The focus of PLT is the client, the impact of any real or perceived event or trauma, regardless of origin, and resolution of the mental, emotional, and physical residue caused by that impact.

Dr. Helen Wambach, psychologist, author, and past-life therapy researcher, conducted small group regressions with several thousand people across the country, suggesting several specific time periods. Following the group regressions, each participant completed a questionnaire regarding such issues as the use of plates and eating utensils, clothing and footwear, type of food consumed, social class, race and sex distribution, and population.[18] She compared details from these group past-life regressions with historical fact, and was amazed at the accuracy of most information gained through regression. Where there was disagreement between her subjects' responses and written historical record, she sought older reference works on the various time periods. She found closer agreement; later volumes had suffered from revision of historical data.

Analyzing the data, she found a surprising correlation between the ratio of males to females in past lives and future lifetimes, and the present-day ratio, which is approximately 49.5 female to 50.5 male. Most of the people in her groups were Caucasian; most in past lives described skin color from black to dark olive with kinky or curly hair, but not straight. Only 10 percent experienced upper-class circumstances in the past.

In her research project, which included future lifetimes as well as past-life experience, Dr. Wambach progressed several thousand people into future time periods, specifically 2100 and A.D. 2300. Only 9 percent of her subjects experienced physical existence in 2100, and only 14 percent experienced physical existence in 2300.

These figures were stable regardless of race or the ratio of males to females in any of the participating groups. Perhaps the results of future-life progressions must be taken seriously because of the statistical analysis of the past-life figures and the accuracy of details of the research that can be verified historically.

Dr. Chet Snow and Dr. Leo Sprinkle continued the work of Dr. Wambach. By 2300, humans will apparently establish colonies in space and carry on routine interaction with extraterrestrials. Snow's book gives an intriguing view of the future of human/ET contact.[19] Our future on Earth will be quite different from present reality, if future-life progressions are valid.

Parallel Lives

There has been much speculation on alternate realities, other dimensions of consciousness, and other planes of spiritual existence. The concept of time seems to be limited to physical existence in a three-dimensional world. In the spirit space, time does not exist and events are simultaneous, as are "lifetimes." Many people can shift focus and spontaneously tap into other lifetimes, past and future, in altered state sessions.[20]

Another speculation regarding consciousness suggests we have several other soul manifestations alive on the planet at present. Not incomplete soul fragments, but aspects of our higher consciousness, the oversoul, each whole and complete. Perhaps analogous to identical twins in the physical realm.

Can we find the others? Can we explore another life in this world? Not an alternate, but a parallel existence, someone we could walk up to and shake hands with? Not a member of our soul family but another aspect of the oversoul? In the altered state, a client can sometimes locate another aspect of themselves. This is an awesome concept.

Regression to Source

Many people suffer feelings of rejection, separation, and abandonment from a partner, family, parents, or friends. This is certainly a common problem that brings people into therapy. It is often described as a pain or emptiness in the heart, or a hole in the gut. Emotions of sadness, grief, confusion, even guilt accompany these sensations. With this combination of emotions and sensations, the bridge inductions are used. The word "feelings" encompasses emotions and physical sensations.

"Let those feelings carry you back. Recall another time you felt the same way in your body. Locate the cause of those feelings. What comes?"

It doesn't take long for clients to uncover a memory of separation from mother in this life. Fortunately, the medical model of birthing has been improved significantly in recent years. More than half of women are still given anesthetic during labor, knocking out the conscious mind. The connection, the feeling of oneness with mother is broken. The newborn infant loses physical, emotional, and psychic contact with mother and interprets this as separation and abandonment.

This is not the first time for the feelings. It is not the origin.

"Let the feelings take you back even farther. Farther back now. Let those feelings take you all the way back. Find the cause of these feelings. Locate the source of the feelings of separation."

Following this suggestion, many clients recall separation from the Creator Source as an individual spark of light. This is the original experience of separation. In the next moment comes a powerful and indescribable memory, the experience just before the separation. This is the experience of oneness with Source before the illusion of separation.

This experience is described by many spiritual disciplines. Many petty concerns disappear, swept away by the magnificence of this moment and the realization of who and what we are really. The ego shrinks from this reality. This is the memory of home, and those who find this place have no doubt of their final destination. We are all going home again. None will be left behind.

Beyond Death

After the death scene in a past-life regression, the newly deceased soul moves toward the Light. The description is similar to accounts of the near-death experience, except the spirit is joined by other beings who come to guide the newcomer all the way into the Light. Only when the newly deceased spirit moves fully into the Light is the past life really over. However, that is only one option for the newly deceased soul.

As the past-life character, through the client's voice, describes the sequence of events following death, it may not perceive the Light. More information is needed on this.

"What happens next?"

Often the narrative leads to a description of "joining" or "coming into" another living person. This is not a past life of the client. This voice is describing the act of spirit possession or attachment. The being who describes this sort of connection has detoured from the ideal path of the reincarnation cycle. A living person cannot be possessed by a past-life personality. Reincarnation is a continuation, not an interruption.

Some describe looking for another body in the hospital, especially the nursery, on the battlefield after death in combat, or just "waiting for another body to come along." Steve, a minister who served as a medic in Vietnam, carried many spirits of men who had died in his arms as he comforted the wounded. As different ones spoke through his voice, they described just "coming up his arms" as they left their bodies. Spirit attachment is a major factor in the condition known as post-traumatic stress disorder.[21]

These descriptions of connecting with another body are not past-life memories of the client; they are recollections of other persons who were attracted to and are attached to the client. These are possessing or attaching entities. In my practice as a past lives therapist, it was disturbing to find so many of my clients describing just such an attachment or attachments (there is never just one attached entity). It was this experience that led me to develop the techniques of spirit releasement therapy.

– 10 –

Spiritualism and the American Society for Psychical Research

Is there life after death? Does the personality survive? Can the spirits of the deceased communicate with living people? The SPR, the Society for Psychical Research, was established in England in 1882 to study these questions. Early work in Spiritualism was conducted with trance mediums, people who have the ability to contact the "spirit world" and communicate with the spirits of the deceased. Spiritualism is based on the belief that human personality survives death intact, and communication with the spirits of the deceased is possible.

Spiritualism began in 1848 in Hydesville, New York, when two young women, the Fox sisters, purportedly received spirit communication in the form of knocking sounds.[1] News of this "spirit communication" spread quickly, and a growing number of people chose to believe these "messages" were from spirits of the deceased. Within two years there were an estimated one hundred "mediums" in New York City. Within a decade, there were millions of believers in the U.S. and in Europe. A new religion had emerged on the human stage: Spiritualism.

Apparently a discarnate entity could incorporate into the medium, taking temporary control or "possession," and would then speak through the medium's voice. Messages for the living would come from a loved one who had died.

Mediumship is defined as the process of a nonphysical intelligent being, usually a discarnate human, that assumes some degree of control of a living person in order to communicate something meaningful. Mediumship is distinguished from the phenomenon of spirit possession in that it occurs only with the deliberate cooperation of the medium and produces a constructive result. The difference is in purpose, duration, and effect.

American Society for Psychical Research

Dr. James Hyslop (1854–1920) was professor of logic and ethics at Columbia University, New York, from 1889 to 1902. He authored a book on psychology in 1895, and taught the subject at Smith College when the science was in its infancy. The points of connection between psychology and parapsychology were not yet clearly drawn.

The American Society for Psychical Research (ASPR) was formed in Boston in 1885. Hyslop was elected president of the ASPR in 1906. Investigation focused on three subjects: the survival of consciousness; spirit obsession, as it was termed then; and multiple personality disorder.

As president of ASPR, Hyslop explored the problem of distinguishing obsession from multiple personality. More than a theoretician, Dr. Hyslop depended on experience and observation of the phenomena he was studying. After he admitted credibility of the existence of spirits, ten years of investigation were required to convince himself of the possibility of obsession by discarnate beings as a cause of mental illness. In the years that followed, he accumulated the facts that make it scientifically probable.[2] He is the pioneer in the systematic investigation of spirit obsession and possession as a cause of mental disorder.

Dr. Carl Wickland was an avowed Spiritualist. Wickland graduated from Durham Medical College in 1900, and nine years later became chief psychiatrist at the National Psychopathic Institute in Chicago. In 1918, he moved to Los Angeles and established the National Psychological Institute, where he continued the work of healing spirit obsession. His seminal work on the treatment of spirit obsession and possession is chronicled in two books, *Thirty Years Among the Dead* (1924) and *Gateway to Understanding* (1934).

Dr. Wickland first became interested in spirit possession after observing the frequency with which people suffered character changes after engaging in such practices as the Ouija board or automatic writing. Many such people required hospitalization for apparent mental illness. Wickland consulted discarnate teachers through his wife, Anna, a gifted medium. He was told that possession of the living by the "Earthbound" spirits of deceased humans was the cause, and that he could alleviate the symptoms of the victims if he followed their instructions. The work was conducted with the help of a "concentration circle," a small group of people assembled to support this rescue work.

Following guidance from the discarnate intelligence, Wickland built a device called a "Wimhurst machine" that generated static electricity. The charges of static electricity from this machine were applied to the head and spine of the afflicted person.

Simultaneously, in another room, Mrs. Wickland was in trance, surrounded by the members of the concentration circle. Mediumistic ability and the trance state are open doors to a discarnate spirit. The entity would disengage from the patient, then incorporate into Mrs. Wickland and begin to speak. The voice would often complain about the "fire" running up the back, referring to the static electricity, and would express annoyance at the disturbance.

Dr. Wickland would converse with the discarnate personality, who would often turn out to be an identifiable deceased person. The first task was to convince the spirit that physical death had occurred and they no longer belonged in the Earth plane. Many spirits are oblivious to the fact that they have died, and are extremely confused concerning their whereabouts. Most of the spirits would quickly grasp the nature of their condition, and would willingly go with the guiding spirits who came for them. The guides often turned out to be loved ones who also had died.[3]

Dr. Hyslop was so impressed with the importance of this type of cure that he established a foundation in his will for the continuance of the work. The James Hyslop Institute was located in New York City, headed by Dr. Titus Bull, a graduate of New York University and Bellevue Medical College. Bull was the first to suggest that one Earthbound spirit could have another Earthbound spirit attached to it as the result of being a victim of obsession before its passing.[4] This describes the nested or layered condition of attached entities often discovered in clinical session.

William James spoke on "Demoniacal Possession" in his 1896 Lowell Lectures. Recapitulating his previous lecture, "Multiple Personality," he mentioned three types of mutations in the sense of self: insane, hysteric, and somnambulistic. The fourth type, he said, is spirit control, or mediumship, which in the past had been equated with devil worship and pathology.

Referring to the spiritualistic activities of Boston and New York in 1896, James stated that the diabolic nature of demon possession now "has with us assumed a benign and optimistic form, [in which] changed personality is considered the spirit of a departed being coming to bring messages of comfort from the 'sunny land.'"[5]

Spiritualism began losing its popularity in 1888 after the public confession by the Fox sisters that they had faked the spirit rappings. Belief in spirit possession became increasingly suspect, and the decline of belief in possession paralleled the decline of interest in multiple personality disorder.

Hypnosis lost favor in professional circles, multiple personality disorder was no longer diagnosed, and the process of exorcism as a healing technique virtually disappeared among the medical practitioners and the clergy as twentieth-century materialism flourished in America.

The Near-Death Experience

Thanks to contemporary medical science, many people have returned from death's door and are able to describe the experience. It seems that consciousness, the personality, the soul, the existential "I" leaves the body, which appears to be "dead" by all medical definitions, moves toward a bright Light, then for any one of many reasons returns to the physical body. For many people this is a vivid and often life-altering experience. The descriptions are amazingly similar, even in other countries and languages.

There is a growing literature on the near-death experience, or NDE.[6] Some people describe recognizing familiar people, though in spirit, and some claim to perceive dark, hostile, even demonic forms. The NDE has been the subject of movies and TV presentations.

After recovering from such an experience, many people can accurately describe events that occurred while the body was clinically dead, including activities of the medical personnel during resuscitation attempts. It seems as if the consciousness separates from the body, remains fully aware and "sees," that is, perceives, everything in the vicinity in precise detail, usually from a vantage point near the ceiling.

Many report being greeted by friends and relatives who are no longer living. Often such people encounter a tunnel and a brilliant Light, and sometimes a figure of religious importance, usually Jesus. At first the Light seems to attract the newly deceased spirit, but at some point the religious figure indicates that it is not yet time, that there is more work to do in the physical body. The spirit of the person then rejoins the body, often much to the surprise of people nearby.

Those who have been resuscitated report that some being or voice told them to return to the body. The Light is so totally peaceful, so indescribably beautiful, that many returnees resent the need to return. It was estimated in 1982 that eight million Americans had gone through the near-death experience.[7] In a later survey, Gallup found that more than eleven million had experienced it.

Some people who die and return report being greeted by friends and relatives no longer living. The implication is that the personality, or soul consciousness, survives physical death as a discrete entity. The term "entity" is defined as an individual consciousness, a whole integral being of distinct and demonstrable existence. By definition, this is a spirit.

This case was described by a skeptical surgeon. A patient died on the operating table as the doctor was working. Several anxious minutes passed before she could be resuscitated. Later, the patient described exactly what the surgical team was wearing, the instruments they were using, what they did to revive her, the equipment in the room, even some accurate details about the adjoining rooms. Physicians often claim such accounts are caused by a toxic drug reaction or hallucination. However, this patient was accurate in the details of her description—*and she was totally blind.* Although still skeptical, the surgeon did acknowledge that something had occurred that was above and beyond his belief systems about reality. Nothing he learned in medical school had prepared him for this.

George Ritchie, a psychiatrist in practice in Virginia, was clinically dead for nine minutes as a result of complications of pneumonia. This occurred while he was a young recruit in Army basic training. During the NDE he was conscious of being out of his body and traveling to many locations.

Among the experiences he described was an episode in a bar. As an out-of-body being, he could perceive discarnate spirits in the bar as well as the living people who were the paying patrons. One drunken man fell to the floor, either dazed or unconscious. Ritchie observed several discarnates rush into his head, apparently through an alcohol-induced weakness in the aura, the protective energy field surrounding the body. He saw the same phenomenon repeated several times during his observation in this location.[8]

NDE and SRT

In a session with Katy, a thirty-one-year-old female client, she described her outbursts of temper and surprisingly foul language. The first entity who emerged was a motorcyclist, rough in character, belligerent toward me, and unwilling to leave. Such unwillingness usually indicates a nested entity within that entity. Deeper probing uncovered a female entity who had attached to him when he was alive and had remained attached. A dark force entity had infiltrated her consciousness and was at the bottom of this nest.

After the transformation of this dark entity, it was released to its appropriate place in the Light. The female entity was then eager to go to the Light. Following this, the biker apologized to Katy, acknowledged that I was not such a bad guy, and agreed to go to the Light.

Katy recalled that some twenty years earlier, as she was driving to the beach to enjoy a day of sun and sand, she had stopped at the scene of a motorcycle accident. She had offered her beach towel to the attending police officer to cover the body of the deceased biker. Her natural compassion was the opening for this guy who died alone on the highway.

With further probing, another spirit emerged. He was a tired old man, not sure about what he was doing with Katy. He recalled and described his experience of dying in a hospital and moving toward the Light. He perceived a young woman approaching him, not from the Light but from the direction of the hospital.

She linked her arm with his and he heard her say, "C'mon, we'll get through this together."

At this point they moved back into her body in tandem. Her natural caring and compassion were the invitation for the attachment. When Katy resumed her normal state of consciousness, she described her very serious gall bladder surgery some years previous. After she recovered, the physicians told her of the severity of her condition, the complicated surgery and the concern they had shared regarding the possibility of her survival and eventual recovery. They had not informed her of any cessation of vital signs. This was her first awareness of her NDE connected with the surgery.

– 11 –

Spirit Releasement Therapy and Past-Life Therapy: Complementary Aspects

At the time of death several choices are available for the deceased soul. It can move into the Light, accompanied by the guiding spirits that come. It can also linger on the Earth plane for any number of reasons, remaining in some favored location as a haunting spirit, or joining a living person as an attached entity.

When a client describes the death scene in a past-life therapy session, the past-life experience is not over and the regression is not complete until the being returns to the Light. If the being does not move toward the Light after death but instead describes floating in a gray place, drifting over their hometown, or being drawn toward a living human, this may indicate a spirit attachment. The therapist continues to probe for the experience of either moving fully into the Light or joining another living person. The discovery questions must continue until one of these two events is recalled.

I continue to repeat my favorite question:

"What happens next?"

The newly deceased spirit may describe a brief period of wandering before moving into the Light. This indicates a past life of the client.

This question may also reveal the experience of attachment to a living host, who is the client. Since a spirit is capable of "floating" indefinitely, more prompting may be needed to locate the crucial moment. The longer the soul remains near the Earth, the more likely is attachment to a living human. The next question is asked:

"Skip forward to the next thing that happens."

This usually uncovers the actual moment when an Earthbound soul joined the living person. Attached entities seldom make their presence known to the host; spirit attachment is usually a surprise to the client. Although the condition of spirit interference is nearly universal, most people are not aware of these parasitic attachments.

During a past-life therapy session, the therapist may intuitively sense that something in the past-life description is not right, and the next question is posed.

"How old was she when you joined her in *this* lifetime?"

If it is a past life of the client, the question will be meaningless and will not interrupt the narrative of past-life events. If an attached entity is speaking, the answer will usually be immediate. The question will catch the entity off guard. It knows it has been discovered. The answer will be given as the age of the host in years or at a certain stage of life.

"She was six."

"He was a baby."

If the answer indicates or suggests infancy, birth, or the prenatal period, the therapist might mistakenly assume the attached entity is the rightful soul of the client. The therapist then asks the question:

"Was there already someone there when you joined?"

This is the clincher. The entity will look again and usually discover the rightful spirit already at home in the body. This means the one speaking through the voice of the client is definitely an attached entity. The attached EB is usually honest and straightforward.

When the condition of a spirit attachment is identified, the releasement can begin. The opportunity for healing is available for two beings, the client and the confused EB.

The following cases are typical of the connection between past-life therapy and spirit releasement therapy, often necessary during sessions.

Diana and the Stone Carver

Diana was thirty-six years old, intelligent and attractive. She wanted to explore the cause of a recurring irritation and tightness in her throat coupled with a fear of unknown but terrible consequences if she dared to speak the truth.

Diana described a previous therapy session in which she had explored a past life in Egypt as a male stone carver working inside a pyramid that was to be the tomb of a pharaoh.

On the day the carvings were finished, the stone carvers were ushered into a small room by three guards. One by one, they were shoved against the wall and their throats cut. This action was taken to prevent them from revealing the nature of the carvings and secret truths they depicted.

This was the source of Diana's fear of the consequences of telling the truth and the tightness and irritation in her throat. However, there was no relief from the condition after that past-life therapy session. This lack of resolution suggests there are traumatic events from other lifetimes contributing to the symptoms. It can also indicate an attached EB imposing the condition. Past-life therapy with an attached entity doesn't seem to bring resolution to the EB or the host/client.

I suggested that Diana focus her awareness on the physical sensation of the irritation in the throat, and go fully into the emotional feelings.

Dr. B.: "If that irritation in your throat could speak, what would it say? If the feelings could talk, what would they say?"

Client: "I can't speak. I can't speak."

The response was emotional and immediate.

Dr. B.: "Say it again. Let the feelings come. Say it again."

By the third repetition of the phrase, she accessed the lifetime and the entire past-life memory, which she had discovered in her earlier session. She continued the story. The stone carver lamented over the lack of time to meditate and prepare for death. As a spirit, he lifted from the body but perceived no Light. He remained in the room.

The therapist must avoid leading questions in a session. Rather, the questions should prompt the narrative without suggesting a direction.

Dr. B.: "What happens next?"

C.: "I'm alone in the room. The guards have removed the bodies. The spirits of the other stone carvers are gone."

Dr. B.: "What happens next?"

The question is repeated gently whenever the unfolding account slows or stops.

The spirit finally moved out of the room, drifted above the town, observed people in the streets, occasionally tampering or interfering with their energy. He was feeling angry. He did not know what to do or where to go.

Dr. B.: "Skip forward to the next thing that happens."

Certain events seem to be more easily recalled. The more emotional energy, the easier the memory is triggered.

Diana jerked in the recliner and began to cry softly.

Dr. B.: "What just happened?"

C.: "He just came into me."

Dr. B.: "How old are you?" The present tense refers to what she had just revealed.

C.: "About thirteen."

Dr. B.: "Stone carver, what happened to you? Do you know this woman? Who is she to you?"

C.: "She wouldn't have anything to do with me. She was married and wouldn't even talk to me. I wanted her."

He was referring to the Egyptian lifetime; he was still focused on his pain and thwarted desire. They were both incarnated at that time, over four thousand years ago. The stone carver was not a past incarnation of Diana, it was an attached entity. He had been Earthbound since the Egyptian lifetime when she rejected him. Unrequited love is a potent force; it kept this stone carver Earthbound more than four millennia while he searched for her.

After his death, he wandered about the area, but did not find her there. He attached to many people before finding Diana in the fullness of her budding femininity in the present lifetime.

In the safe space of the session, he was able to express his anger and resentment at her rejection of him in that lifetime. Beneath that was his love for her. Finally he realized he could not be with her in the way he wanted as long as he remained connected in this way. He still wanted her, and clearly had plans for their future together. He eagerly moved into the Light with the spirit helpers who came for him.

Nested Entities

Nancy was a thirty-six-year-old psychotherapist. She wanted to experience past-life therapy and chose to work on her drinking problem. She spoke about waking night after night at about three in the morning to take "a couple of belts" of Scotch before being able to sleep again. She mentioned other aspects of her problem, but the use of the terminology "a couple of belts" was not in keeping with her lovely feminine nature.

As she continued to talk about the drinking, I asked if she felt any sensations in her body as she spoke. She described a feeling of nausea in her stomach. As she focused on the sensation, she began to see swirling shapes of yellow and orange color. Suddenly there emerged the scene of a saloon. A cowboy stood drinking at the bar. His name was Tom. He was a heavy drinker. Married to a woman who despised him for this excess, he slept in a separate bedroom. Routinely he took his bottle of whiskey to bed and would take a couple of belts before falling asleep.

Tom, through Nancy, told of many occasions, including his daughter's wedding, when he overindulged and his wife would send him away from the house. He was always glad to be away. Late one night at home in his own bed, he began to feel pain in his stomach. He took a few more belts of whiskey to ease the pain, but the feeling spread across his belly until he felt like his guts were on fire.

The pain and nausea were so bad he called to his wife to go for the doctor. She angrily refused, which infuriated him, and he had some foul things to say about women. He died that night in pain, drunk and angry at women. He likely had a perforated ulcer through which the whiskey seeped, spreading to the tender tissues within the abdomen.

Intuitively, I felt this was not a past-life memory of Nancy's. The next question is used if an attached entity is suspected.

Dr. B.: "Tom, how old was Nancy when you joined her?"

C.: "She was fourteen and she was having an argument with her father."

The answer came immediately, without hesitation.

Dr. B.: "Tom, was there ever a time in your life when you felt like something just came into you and took over?"

C.: "Yes, I was sixteen and I was having an argument with my father."

There was surprise in his voice as he realized what had happened. This is the kind of similarity that often attracts an EB.

Dr. B.: "Is that other one still here? Is the person who entered Tom still here?"

After only a brief hesitation, Nancy's voice said softly:

C.: "Yes."

At the end of the session she revealed that her clearest mental imagery of the entire session was at the moment that Tom recalled the feeling of being entered.

Dr. B.: "What's your name?"

C.: "Larry." Nancy's voice was matter-of-fact.

Dr. B.: "Larry, what happened?"

C.: "I was working in the assay office and they accused me of stealing gold. They were real mad at me so I left there. I had a bottle of whiskey I was drinking. I was walking along the railroad track and a train hit me."

He died drunk and angry. Did he impose his habits and attitudes on Tom? Seems like more than a coincidence.

Dr. B.: "Well, Larry, did you steal it?"

After a pause he admitted the truth:

C.: "Yes."

Larry sounded so tired. He responded to the description of the Light and was immediately ready to leave. Guiding spirits appeared and lovingly assisted him on his journey home.

Tom was relieved to discover and release this entity nested within himself. After a parting dialogue with Nancy, he eagerly accompanied the guides who came for him.

An Accidental Connection

Are accidents really accidents? Coincidence and synchronicity offer a fascinating field of investigation. Depth psychologist Carl Jung suggested that synchronicity could be defined as "meaningful coincidence." Jung described a case of a young woman patient who resisted his therapeutic efforts. She had an excellent education, arming her with a staunch rationalism that controlled her view of reality.

The patient related an impressive dream in which someone had given her a golden scarab—a costly piece of jewelry. At the same moment, Jung heard something tapping on the window behind him. It was a fairly large flying insect. He opened the window and caught the insect in his hand as it flew into the darkened room. It was a common rose-chafer, a scarabaeid beetle whose gold-green color resembles that of a golden scarab. He handed the beetle to the patient with the words, "Here is your scarab." This incident punctured her normal rational exterior, and therapy was able to proceed with satisfactory results.[1]

A female client of mine, in her sixties and retired from the Panama Canal Company, discovered a young male EB in her space. He had been a sailor on a supply ship in the early 1900s during the construction of the canal. He died of malaria and just stayed around, eventually drifting into a house a few miles south of the Canal Zone. Over the decades, the house gained the reputation of being haunted.

The client and a few friends often drove up into the countryside for Sunday picnics. One of the group was a young American sailor on a naval ship stationed in the Canal Zone. The EB perceived the young man driving the car and decided to attach so he could do the things young sailors do since he had died so young. He "zoomed" out of the house toward the car, shot past the driver, and collided with the woman in the passenger seat, where he became stuck. He was frustrated in his desire to lead the carefree, libertine life as she, our client, was conservative in her habits. He was more than ready to leave her to go to the Light and start over again.

Was this attachment accidental? Is there perfect order in our spiritual universe, or is it random?

In my spiritual worldview, randomness left me feeling somehow unsafe and unprotected. I longed for perfect order. In my first years of discovering and learning about discarnate interference, I questioned attached entities at great length, guiding them to recall some connection with the host, whether in past lives, the spirit realm between lives, or possible future existence. About half the attached entities have no other interaction with the host, no past-life connection or unfinished business. No karmic bond, no prior agreement existed. It's just a matter of being in the wrong place at the wrong time. Such randomness can be unsettling.

The Holocaust

The events surrounding the Holocaust represent the darkest period of our recent history. This terrible energy continues to impact the spiritual paths of millions of beings: those whose lives ended without explanation in death camps; the survivors who lost loved ones there; and the German citizens who were pulled unwillingly or unwittingly into the maelstrom that was Nazi Germany.

The Holocaust still burns painfully in the minds and memories of many people, even through the time buffer of more than half a century. The reality of a Nazi hoard of gold hidden in Swiss banks, gold from jewelry and gold extracted from the teeth of the Jewish victims of the death camps, continues to be a highly contentious and emotionally charged issue.

Only recently did a group of Swiss banks, in a reluctant validation of the allegations, offer a settlement of $600 million. The World Jewish Congress refused this offer as insufficient, claiming at least twice that much is due the death camp survivors and their families. Either amount seems an insult in the face of the human suffering and unimaginable personal violations that allowed the accumulation of the gold which in part financed the last years of the Nazi war machine.

Many people living today, Jewish and non-Jewish, have recalled past lives as Jews in Germany during the nightmare of World War II.[2] Clients have described placing on their door frame the *mezuzah*, a small case containing a parchment inscribed with Deuteronomy 6:4–9 and 11:13–21 and the name *Shaddai*, a sign and reminder of the Jewish faith, even though many are not Jewish by birth or faith.

Some have described an inexplicable attraction to the traditions and rituals of Judaism and feeling strangely at home in a synagogue.

Some seem to have a familiarity with Jewish history and customs, an affinity with Jewish people, even an urge to travel to Germany. These identification points are not disturbing, just curious to people who uncover such memories and feelings.

What is disturbing to clients in an altered state is a past-life memory of being Jewish in Nazi Germany. They recall being arrested by the Gestapo, brutalized, separated from family members, herded aboard trains and trucks, and transported to the camps. The memories seem real, the atrocities committed there palpable. Clients often recognize present family members as being in the camps with them.

Anorexia nervosa is a disorder usually occurring in teenage women, characterized by an abnormal fear of becoming obese, a distorted self-image, a persistent aversion to food, and severe weight loss. All anorexics are dominated by their fears of violating rituals.[3]

The physical appearance of the anorexic woman is familiar to anyone who has seen photos of survivors of the death camps at the time of liberation. Emaciation is extreme, the appearance of muscle wasting and bulging skeletal joints reveals the clear evidence of starvation.

Manipulative behavior, typical of the anorexic, and the fear of violating ritual may be related to unconscious memories of survival in these camps and attempts to gain some semblance of control in the situation, however illusory that might have been. Morris Netherton, author of *Past Lives Therapy,* has described cases from his practice in which clients discovered lifetimes in the Nazi death camps. He has successfully treated anorexia through past-life therapy.[4]

Historical records indicate there were some favorites among the women prisoners, those who were used for the sexual pleasure and perversion by the Nazi guards.

Trini

Trini, a female client, uncovered a past-life memory from a death camp. She was a sexual favorite until one night when she was taken to a secluded cave near the camp and tortured to death in a satanic worship ritual. Severe soul fragmentation resulted from the torture and threats to remove her female organs and keep those parts captive there in the cave. In her distressed state, she fully believed the threats. As a spirit, she watched as they fulfilled the threat and removed her reproductive organs, placing them in a large glass container.

In the session, the DFEs were released, as the first step in therapy. The soul fragmentation was recovered after clarifying the misperceptions and correcting false beliefs. Following this, the past-life work led to resolution and forgiveness.

More frequent than uncovering past-life memories in the death camps is discovery of attached entities of the tortured souls of those who died there. Many people who suffer such trauma remain Earthbound following death, continuing to suffer the emotional and physical pain of their unspeakable ordeal. In some cases, the living host for these Earthbound entities reincarnated after dying in the camps. Entities often attach to someone who survived, or a family member who was born long after the war ended. These family bonds are extremely close.

Sarina

Sarina believed she had lived in Nazi Germany during the war. She had some memories of the camp and repetitive images of elbows and backs of heads as if she were being herded along with many other people. She had no idea of the layout of the camp, no awareness of what happened to anyone but her.

In that persona, she knew nothing of the immense horror of the network of camps across Germany and beyond. She had no memory of anything following her death in the camp, nothing about going to the Light, preparing for rebirth, or a present-life experience. During sessions with another past-life therapist, that persona had emerged several times and had spoken, actually forming a friendship with the therapist. He began to suspect an attached entity rather than a past life and referred her to us.

In the session, the entity emerged almost immediately and identified itself as her grandfather, whom she never knew. Apparently, some family members had escaped from Germany while it was still possible. The grandfather had died shortly after arriving at a camp.

As with millions of family tragedies in that time, no one ever heard of him again. This kind of unfinished business, the terrible unknowing, and the incompletion of never having said good-bye, weighed heavily on the family for decades. Surviving family members were currently planning a memorial service as a family completion for the would-have-been patriarch whom most of them had never known.

During the session, Sarina asked him questions, shared her feelings with him, and seemed to resolve much of her own anxiety and depression. In a loving farewell, she released him into the Light he had not known. She was eager to share her experience with her family, even though some would think it weird. At the completion of the session, Sarina felt an inner peace she had been seeking for years.

Marian

Marian was appalled to learn that she had died in a Nazi death camp. She discovered several attached entities of children who described their short existence in the camp. When their mothers were sent to the ovens, these children had gathered around teenaged Marian, and they called her their caretaker. As they described the scene, she recalled the events with horror. In her present reincarnation the Earthbound souls of these children found their caretaker again and attached themselves to her.

David

David experienced an upsetting emotional reaction during a lecture on spirit releasement therapy, so he scheduled an appointment. He uncovered a prior existence in a Nazi death camp. He had not been very old when he died. With further investigation, he discovered the entity of his mother from that lifetime who had died before him in the camp and had attached to him immediately. She reattached to him in the present lifetime. Both had been subjected to medical experimentation, which led to their deaths.

Next he discovered the attached entity of the German medical doctor who had conducted the crude procedures. The doctor claimed that he suffered such guilt, he had taken his own life. That ended nothing but his physical body, and he was compelled to attach to the boy, along with mother. Apparently many German physicians cast a blind eye to behaviors of their colleagues as well as their own deeds during this period. The unspoken yet clearly understood dictate of the time was "follow orders or die."

After processing the memories and the all-important forgiveness experience, the doctor and mother were ready to release and move into the Light. I requested the mother to look deeper and explore for other attachments with David. As she looked, her voice suddenly tightened with fear; she perceived a terrifying darkness. She had discovered the DFEs attached to her son. I asked if she would prefer to move on, and she quickly agreed. Along with the doctor, she moved into the safety of the Light.

The focus of the session shifted to the DFEs with David, the darkness in the camp, and beyond to the dark influence within the Nazi hierarchy. In every such session, many DFEs are uncovered and released. We request Archangel Michael to expose and dismantle the dark networks involved, and the oppressive darkness of that episode in history is diminished. Before David's session ended, many DFEs were released. He was astonished. The dark circles beneath his eyes softened and lightened immediately.

The Third Reich was rife with dark force energy, from the Nazi flag of red and black, the signal colors of the DFEs, to the fierce aggression on European neighbors, to the subjugation and ethnic cleansing of the Jewish people. Hitler actively courted the demonic forces. He was a man completely obsessed by his desire for power. This aspect of his life and dramatic rise to political power is well documented.[5]

Some people suggest that Hitler was the Antichrist, bent on ruling the world, and the prophesies of the Book of Revelation are being played out as written. In this reality, however, there was defeat of the darkness, though at great cost in material resources as well as human suffering. And the cleanup continues.

In many therapy sessions, the client can locate no association in this or a former life with such an entity. No Jewish connection can be found. The attachment is random.

When we find attached entities who died in the death camps, if the client is willing, we proceed with a group remote spirit releasement for the Earthbound souls still imprisoned in the camps. This is rescue work on a grand scale. In their anguish, their focus remains on the morass of emotions, the tangle of bodies, the stench and filth in the camps.

Attached entities describe the "showers" that were actually gas chambers. As they rise from their physical bodies sprawled on the floor of the chambers, they see others rising up and mingling with many more who have gathered there. Bodies are removed and more people are shoved into the rooms. As these succumb to the lethal gas, their souls also rise to join the growing mass of entities floating there. Few seem to leave that place on their own.

Entities give similar descriptions of the ovens where people were burned alive, as entities group together unable to leave the enclosure. The terror is personal, the compassion is generalized to others. In their pain and confusion they cling together, stuck in the location of their death.

Many were forced to dig mass graves, long pits in the ground, before being shot and buried. Some were buried alive after being shot and only wounded. Children were buried without being shot, not considered worthy of wasting a bullet. Some of these entities are still lodged in the dirt, many are discovered floating about the grounds, yet within the camp boundaries.

Along with Earthbound souls imprisoned in the camps, the emotional residue of rage, terror, grief, guilt, anguish, and confusion hangs like a dense fog, a funereal pall over the death scenes. Extensive spiritual cleansing is required.

Some guards also died there, by natural causes, suicide, by execution following disobedience, or at the hands of the prisoners. Absolute discipline also applied to the camp guards, many of whom were young soldiers, decent men who could not countenance the excesses of the Nazi regime. They are also Earthbound in these dark places, burdened with fear and guilt.

The attached entities nearly always accept the offer to assist in remote rescue work. Time as we experience it does not exist for spirits; the suffering continues unabated to this day. There is a tremendous inflow of light as we begin the remote work. The entity describes the inside of the gas chamber, oven, or the mass grave.

They call out to the hovering, wailing masses of Earthbound souls, who are dazed and at first unresponsive, frozen in their confusion. As the Light comes, the lost souls begin to move. Disbelief changes to acceptance.

Many of these entities immediately grasp what is happening, and they guide others toward the Light. Some need intense urging. Many who died in the camps have found their way to the Light. These beings come to assist in the rescue, along with many light beings. It is a holy moment.

This remote rescue work has also be done for locations such as the Holocaust Memorial Museum in Washington, D.C. From the results of direct releasement work, we can trust that remote spirit releasement is also effective. It is a privilege to be part of such an exodus.

DFEs and Nested Entities

In most sessions, we find EBs attached to clients. Many were held Earthbound following their death by other EBs attached to them. They simply could not go to the Light after death. This nesting of entities sometimes appears to have dozens of layers.

When we explore this nested situation, we often find the innermost entity is a dark force entity, the classic demon. I began this work without any belief in spirits, spirit possession, and certainly no belief in demonic possession. However, in the course of working with thousands of people, I have discovered this type of entity to be common. I don't like what I've learned about spirit interference in general and the activities of such DFEs in particular.

After discovering this type of being in many sessions, I began reading the classic religious literature on possession by demonic spirits and the classic procedures of exorcism and deliverance ministry. There seemed to be more than a little truth in the old literature and in some of the newer books by Christian fundamentalists.

The DFEs may serve spiritual evolution as a "thrust block," a starting point from which a being can choose in favor of the Light. The choice between Light and Dark is arguably the most important choice a conscious being can make. Possibly, Light and the Dark are polarities of the same energy that allows human beings to exercise the gift of free will.

Through years of practice, information about the process of discarnate interference, the effects of spirit attachment, and the descriptions of the dark force entities and their behavior has been consistent. People are describing something that is universal in human experience. The spirit releasement work has been done in other countries in many languages. Techniques of past-life therapy and spirit releasement therapy have brought profound results in our clients. Many therapists use these techniques with similar success. I have come to accept the validity of the spiritual reality as described by many thousands of people.

– 12 –
Spirit Attachment or Past Life?

Many traditional therapists and counselors reject the idea of past-life therapy, partly because it is based on the controversial spiritual notions of reincarnation and karma. Most traditional therapists and many past-life therapists reject the concept of spirit releasement therapy because it is based on the objectionable and, to many, frightening possibility of spirit possession.

Spirit releasement therapy and past-life therapy are closely linked in clinical practice. The event that led to the spirit attachment is often discovered in a past life of the client. This must be explored through the techniques of PLT. The past-life events described and experienced by a client may be part of the soul memory not of that client, but of an attached entity. Differential diagnosis is critically important, the identity of the one speaking must be established before the appropriate techniques can be followed.

Past-life therapy is so effective in so many problem situations, it is a surprise when it doesn't work well. PLT on a discarnate entity accomplishes little to nothing toward relief of the problem affecting the client. The therapist often can't tell which condition, past-life trauma or attached entity, is present until well into the session. The following reports demonstrate the connection between past-life therapy and spirit releasement therapy in cases of physical and psychological problems.

Eating Disorder

Gayle, a thirty-five-year-old female client, suffered with bulimia, an eating disorder involving eating binges followed by self-induced vomiting, use of laxatives, and other efforts to control weight. She had been bulimic for twenty-one years, beginning at age fourteen. Since that time, she had gone through the binge-purge eating cycle three times a day on average—a very severe case. In the discovery process, I directed Gayle to locate the source of the condition.

The character that emerged was a woman who had died one hundred years earlier. She had killed her deformed Siamese twin children, then escaped into the woods outside of town, successfully eluding the authorities for the remainder of her life. She would sneak into town at night, eating whatever she could and as much as she could. She also ate whatever she could find in the woods.

Past-life memory? Could be. However, I suspected an entity. I asked the question:

"How old was Gayle when you joined her in this lifetime?"

If it is a past life of the client, the question is meaningless and the client will ignore it. If it is an entity, it will answer immediately. This one did.

When she was fourteen and suffering from typical teenage female emotional stress, the entity joined her, urging her to:

". . . eat, eat, it will make you feel better."

The initial intention of the entity was to be helpful to the girl. However, Gayle gained considerable weight and was unhappy about it. The entity then urged her to:

". . . throw up, it will make you feel better."

The entity was asked to follow that thought back to where it began. Gayle was sitting cross-legged on the floor with a box of tissue in front of her. Good thing. She suddenly began to retch; she clutched her abdomen and doubled over in pain. Her head landed in the box of tissue. The entity apparently had eaten some poison berries that had made her ill. Vomiting eased her pain, and made her "feel better."

This was the genesis of the binge-purge cycle that the spirit of the woman from another time had imposed on this girl in the classic pattern of bulimia. The entity was happy to find peace by going to the Light.

Gayle was immediately relieved of the compulsion to binge and purge. Several months later the referring therapist, who had observed the session, reported that the client was bingeing and purging perhaps two to three times per week, but with no real power behind the act. It seemed to be just a nagging habit and no longer a compulsion. They worked on this in her ongoing therapy.

Sleep Disorder

Randy was a flight attendant, young and handsome. He had chosen a gay lifestyle, yet had little success making a relationship work. Often in his sleep he would kick his partner out of bed. Randy had a fear of going to sleep. Even in infancy and childhood, Randy had feared sleeping. He would kneel or stand with his hands on the edge of the crib, rocking back and forth, shaking the entire crib. As an adult, he would hold on to the foot of his bed and rock in the same manner.

He knew and had always known that this behavior would keep the "thing" in the room away from him, and he would be safe. In therapy, he was achieving good results in areas other than his nighttime behavior. Frustrated in her efforts, his therapist referred him to me for an exploration of spirit attachment.

Randy went easily into the altered state, and he was directed to locate the source of the behavior. Living in Rome during the first century A.D., he had adopted a gay lifestyle, yet kept it hidden from his family. Occasionally he met his lover in a small apartment at the edge of the town where he lived. One night, Randy went to the apartment, unaware that his lover was already there, asleep. Startled at the noise of Randy's entrance, the lover, fearful in his sleepy state, grabbed his spear and killed the "intruder," which turned out to be his beloved.

This traumatic experience in a past life would be accepted by most past-life therapists as the easy explanation of his sleep disorder and fear of the "thing" in the room. Yet there was more. The lover, distraught and horrified by his deed, took his own life. His guilt and remorse kept him Earthbound. He joined Randy early in this life-time as an attached entity; his own memories and emotions blended with Randy's. From this combination of past-life trauma and attached entity developed the sleep disorder and the fear of the "thing" in the room.

The lover perceived the inappropriateness of the situation. He was quick to release his guilt and remorse, and replace it with love. He moved into the Light to happily await the reunion with Randy after completion of his life span on Earth.

I received a glowing report from his therapist a few months later. Randy was sleeping well, and his therapy was going much better than before the session.

Sexual Orientation

Sexual orientation may be an inborn characteristic. Many gay people describe knowing without doubt from a young age they were "different." Approaching sexual maturity, they were drawn to same-sex interaction. For them, it is natural, not a crime, not a mental ill-ness, and not an aberration.

For some, same-sex relationships are a matter of choice. Some people are simply curious and have no hesitation to enjoy sensual pleasures with both sexes. For them, the usual boundaries on sexual activity don't exist. The term "bisexual" has been suggested for this outlook. It may or may not be valid.

A male client described his small-town life and naiveté as a youth. Not until his senior year in college did he hear classmates talking about lesbianism. He asked the meaning of the term and was shocked. His response: "Why would anyone want to do that?" However, in personality tests of his male/female balance, he had always scored about 99 percentile toward the feminine. He is sensi-tive, compassionate, and is a gifted psychological counselor. He is decidedly heterosexual.

One client described his foray into homosexual activity. After his divorce from his first wife, he hated women so much, he falsely assumed he must be homosexual. He tried it for two weeks, realized his attitude toward his former wife had nothing to do with his sexual preferences, and resumed what was, for him, normal interaction with women.

Several female inmates in a prison where I volunteered as a hypnotherapist stated flatly that in prison they chose other women as partners because they were lonely for intimacy and sexual pleasure. It was clearly a matter of choice in those circumstances. After release from incarceration, they knew they would go right back to heterosexual relationships.

It seems there are many choices and predilections involved in sexual orientation and interaction. However, an attached entity of the opposite gender can cause confusion over gender orientation and sexual behavior. This confusion can lead to homosexuality, transvestism, or transsexualism, and gender reassignment surgery. Many people who are unhappy with their sexual orientation and want to change have been freed of these behaviors after releasing the entity that caused what was, for them, a problem.

Gender Dysphoria

Frank was fifty-five. He had been a transvestite for fifty years. He first became fascinated with his mother's underwear when five years old. During his preteen and teen years, he stole articles of women's clothing from clotheslines in his neighborhood, eventually collecting enough to have his own female wardrobe. His wife knew of his condition, but his grown children did not. He was a strong man, masculine to the point of macho, not delicate in any way. He worked in a demanding, forceful position as a personnel recruiter. The attached entity was a woman who had been his baby-sitter when a young child. She had died in a trolley accident.

By the next day after the session, Frank said he felt like a new man, as if a ten-ton weight had been lifted out of his guts. After three months, he was certain that she, the entity, and the urge to wear feminine clothing were gone. He "wanted to shout it from the rooftops." Four months after the session he reported that it was back. He was again enjoying dressing as a woman and this was depressing for him. Two weeks later, he described this brief episode as only a passing fancy. It was gone again.

Six months later he was still free of the practice and yet could remember the excitement and pleasure derived from wearing the feminine attire. They were now stored in trunks in his garage.

Following the session, I received a letter from his wife. Though she loved him and tolerated the fetish, it had bothered her a great deal. Things had changed, she wrote, and she praised the session as the most significant event in their seven-year marriage.

I have worked with several male preoperative transsexuals. After the release of the dominating female entities, they experienced a complete reversal of the desire for gender reassignment.

Hal, a sixty-two-year-old architect, chose to keep the female entity we discovered. He attributed his artistic ability to her influence. Releasement is never forced and is the client's choice. The entity claimed to be Shirley, a girlhood friend of his mother who had died in a boating accident on Lake Michigan several years before his birth. She had entered and attached to him at about the sixth or seventh week in utero. His mother had called him Shirley during the entire prenatal period.

Still troubled with the gender dysphoria, he sought therapy with a female psychologist who also understood the concept of spirit influence, but only had limited knowledge of spirit releasement procedures. During the first session she discovered and released the entity immediately when it manifested. She asked Hal to visualize an apple orchard, then she sent the entity into the orchard. She did not ask his permission.

The next morning he called me to report that for the first time in his life, he had awakened "not confused." Before that morning he had not known what it was like to be single-minded. He had nothing with which to compare his mental state since Shirley had been with him prior to birth.

Sitting in church three days later, Hal, lulled by the sermon, was staring at a mother-of-pearl necklace around the neck of a woman seated nearby. His mind drifted. Suddenly he felt a whooshing sensation; the spirit of the female apparently returned.

Hal chose to allow her to remain and he continued to see another therapist in an attempt to solve his gender dysphoria through conventional sex therapy. Several years later he was still feeling the urge to cross-dress and still considering gender reassignment surgery. He was sixty-eight years old and newly married. For a while in this marriage, he maintained his old apartment, occasionally dressing as a woman. His new wife accepted this, though she did not like it.

Within months, he let his apartment go, fully involving himself in marriage and family life. He still thought about Shirley, felt her presence, and missed the feeling of dressing as a beautiful woman. Even after several years of marriage, he still thought about dressing in female attire. Still in therapy for the gender dysphoria, he refused to release Shirley. He stated that if anything happened to the marriage, he would not rule out gender reassignment surgery.

Burnout

Jolene was a thirty-four-year-old nurse suffering from "burnout." During the four-hour midday drive from her home to the session, she had to stop several times for short naps. This is a type of spirit-induced resistance and is not uncommon. The spirit attempts to divert the client, either by inducing a lapse of memory of appointment times, causing illness, or causing sleep, as in this case. In her weekly routine, the woman hated to go to work and was barely able to trudge up the steps of the hospital. This situation had gradually worsened.

The first of many attached entities to be discovered was the spirit of an angry sixteen-year-old girl who had died of leukemia in the hospital. She hovered over the door of her room, unaware she could leave through walls or the ceiling. The next person to enter the room following her death was Jolene, and the entity immediately attached.

My first session with Jolene lasted six hours. Two days later, the second session lasted two hours. Many discarnates were released. The woman, once again, was happy with her work.

Spirit attachment is a typical cause of burnout, especially with nurses. Usually committed to their profession, they are compassionate and empathetic with patients. Caring is often the magnet that draws spirits of patients who die in the hospital.

Chronic Fatigue Syndrome

Susan was in her late thirties, attractive, intelligent, an attorney no longer practicing her profession. She had lost her husband by suicide several years earlier, and she still felt the loss deeply. In that same year, she had undergone a life-threatening surgery. There were many opportunities for spirit attachment and fragmentation of consciousness.

Several years prior to our session, Susan had uncovered memories of sexual abuse by her father at the age of six. He had raped her more than once. Certainly it was a forbidden subject within the family. Unfortunately, her parents lived only a few miles from her, and she was required to see them occasionally on a social basis. Since discovering the abuse, this interaction was a terrible ordeal for her.

Through conversation with siblings, she discovered her older sister, a psychologist, had also suffered the same torture. Susan was severely depressed, and physically exhausted. Even more devastating for her, she had lost her connection with what she termed her inner Christ.

Typically, she would arise in the morning, perform whatever few tasks needed doing, then return to bed before noon. Susan suffered from chronic fatigue syndrome (CFS), and there seemed to be no conventional treatment available. She had considered suicide more than once during the prior several years. There remained little purpose in life for her.

Susan learned of past-life therapy by seeing psychiatrist Brian Weiss, M.D., on TV, and decided to try it. Why not? Nothing else had worked. With a waiting list of several years, Dr. Weiss referred her to another psychiatrist when she called his office. An appointment was scheduled. Under hypnosis, Susan was directed to locate the cause of her debilitating CFS.

Immediately she recalled the first rape scene at the age of six. While she was in the throes of this traumatic memory, the psychiatrist abruptly interrupted her with the statement (paraphrased from her memory):

"You'll have to handle that yourself, I don't deal with childhood sexual abuse trauma. I only do past-life therapy."

This was a serious clinical error, worsened by an unfeeling attitude on the part of a mental health professional. As a self-proclaimed past-life therapist, he also committed a conceptual error. Rarely does anything begin in the present lifetime. This painful childhood episode most certainly echoed a traumatic event in a prior life. Clearly, the psychiatrist missed the opportunity to heal unfinished business from an earlier lifetime.

She left his office in a seriously suicidal state. Her sister urged a malpractice suit; she refused.

We received an urgent call from Susan. The sister knew of our work and referred her to us. During the first session, we succeeded in releasing a number of layers of dark force entities. They were harvesting the energy of her anguish and blocking any emotional progress she might have made. Removal of the layered dark entities was necessary before the personal issues could be addressed. There was severe fragmentation of consciousness, but she did not have the strength to continue working that day. She felt only slight relief after the session.

A few days later, we conducted a remote session, requested by Susan, and released more attached entities and recovered much of the soul fragmentation. Susan reported a tremendous boost in her energy level, and her will to live. Recovery had begun.

In her next session, she again chose to seek the source of the CFS. Memory of the sexual trauma came up immediately. Along with the memory came the terror and the awful questions:

"Why? Why did he do this? It hurts so much, why don't I die? What have I done to deserve this?"

The bridge inductions assisted her in uncovering the past-life trauma. She, as a man, had been a follower of Jesus. Political leaders of the time deemed this a crime, and he was arrested, imprisoned, and beaten unmercifully, though not severely enough to cause death. Allowed to recover, he was questioned about Jesus and His teachings, urged to renounce Him, and again severely beaten when he refused.

The grinding agony of the questions continued:

"Why? Why is he doing this? It hurts so much, why don't I die? What have I done to deserve this?"

This pain, this fear, and the unanswered questions, were part of the unfinished business that Susan carried from the first century into the present life. The third time he was beaten, he succumbed. In that place of no pain, disconnected from the body, we processed the event. She recognized her torturer in that life as her father in the present life. She compared the fear, the pain, and the unanswered questions, and found both situations to be identical in context.

Reliving the earlier torture and death brought some understanding of the interaction, some unraveling of the connecting threads, yet failed to bring resolution of the question, "Why?"

Two avenues of exploration were now available: to find the connecting event, the other side of the coin so to speak, the earlier episode that had set the forces in motion leading to the beating death and the sexual abuse; or to explore for an external element, either a force or a being, that had influenced the stream of events. The latter is a necessary part of therapy and is often more rapid in bringing resolution.

Dr. B.: "From where you are, above the body, look into the eyes of the torturer. What do you perceive?"

C.: "Anger. He's so angry."

Dr. B.: "What color do you see in his eyes?"

C.: "They're red. Just angry and red."

This is a sure sign of the demonic at work. Jesus wasn't just a teacher. He was a major threat to the forces of darkness, to their plan on Earth, to their activities as they enjoyed free rein among humans who could not see them and denied their existence. The situation is essentially the same today.

The dark beings were intent on suppressing the teachings and breaking or destroying all those who were listening. A dark force network was focused on the followers of Jesus. It still operates, along with many other dark force networks attempting to block any form of teaching of Light.

Susan was directed to look at her father's eyes during the rape episode. She saw the same red eyes. The same dark beings had infested her father in his incarnations over the centuries, standard operating procedure for dark force entities and dark networks.

This red-eyed DFE and its underlings were released simultaneously from torturer and father: a remote spirit releasement for father in the present and for the torturer nearly two thousand years ago. Relief was palpable in the room. We were silent.

With this completion, Susan was finally willing that forgiveness could occur between herself and her father. In this session, she found answers to the question: "Why?" She was able to replace the earlier questions with the statement:

C.: "Forgiveness is the key to healing."

Later she reported that her father was acting differently toward her. He had changed immediately after the remote spirit releasement. Her attitude toward him had changed also, and she was feeling a deep sense of peace about him.

Repeated incarnation in human form provides opportunities to resolve, heal, and forgive everyone, including ourselves, who have been involved in traumatic events of the past. It seems we will bring up the same unresolved issues time after time, lifetime after lifetime, until healing and forgiveness are completed. Issues can take new forms, such as the death at the hands of a Roman torturer in an earlier lifetime and rape by a father in this life. Both exemplify the core issue of victimhood.

The being who was both torturer and father/abuser took on the detestable role of child molester in this life to bring Susan the opportunity of resolving and forgiving. There may have been many intervening lifetimes when the core issue was brought up and she did not manage to bring completion to the issue.

This is an aspect of reincarnation that cannot be overlooked. As past-life therapists, we see this mechanism operating so well. Without this introspection, processing, and completion, the same core issue might emerge in countless future incarnations.

One more thing remained that Susan wanted to accomplish. She wanted to reconnect with that part of the Oneness that is herself. She did. In the next session, she rediscovered the Christ of her being. This was a deeply personal and profoundly spiritual accomplishment. It was a privilege for us to share it.

Children and SRT

Children are not immune to spirit attachment. They can experience strong emotional reactions, much as adults. In their innocence, they are easy targets for opportunistic entities. The spirit of a child who was molested can join a child who is being molested. A lonely child is like a magnet to the spirit of a nanny or governess.

Twelve-year-old Juli came into session with her mother, Jana. The child exhibited the annoying habit of clinging to her mother. It was most bothersome at night, when the girl begged the mother not to leave her bedside, and in the mornings when her mother delivered Juli to school. With the car double-parked and other motorists impatient, Juli would beg her mother to stay just a little longer. Her oft-repeated plea was:

"Mama, please don't go."

Jana had heard of my work and wanted to know if past-life therapy could help her daughter. I briefly explained the process to them and also the concept of spirit attachment. Jana was willing to try anything, and Juli agreed.

In session, Juli and her mother were sitting side by side. Juli quietly watched her mother as she described her daughter's behavior, a plaintive expression on her face. I chose to try the direct approach. With a client in the altered state, especially a heightened emotional state, this often brings an immediate response if an entity is attached.

I asked:

"Is there someone else here with Juli? Is there someone else in Juli's body? If there is someone else here with Juli, what is the first thing that one would say?"

There was no verbal response from Juli when this direct approach was used. There were some body sensations, but there was no coherent conversation. Another induction was needed. I directed her to recall and describe a situation during which she felt fear when mother was leaving.

She told of a recent incident when she felt the familiar anxiety. As she did, the feelings grew more intense. She turned toward her mother, got up on her knees on the couch, and put both arms around her. This was an expression of stark fear as Juli manifested the clinging behavior that so irritated her mother. This could have been the recall of a past-life traumatic memory. I used the affect bridge age regression induction.

"Juli, recall another time when you felt like that. Let those feelings take you back to another time you felt the same way. Let your mind go back to another time when you felt scared just like this."

She turned back and sat down. Her head immediately tipped over onto the back of the couch.

Juli recalled a past life in which she was a fifteen-year-old boy, and her mother, Jana, was a fifteen-year-old girl. The boy was standing in a meadow and the girl, whom he described as "his love," was walking away from him, her family having forbidden the romance. He didn't speak with her again until the day he died.

He never stopped loving her and never married. On his deathbed he received a visit from the woman, his first since they were fifteen. She professed her lifelong love for him, and her sorrow at the social differences that had prevented their union. As she walked away, he begged her not to leave:

"Please, don't go!"

The woman did not turn back. He died shortly thereafter, bereft at her leaving.

This could be a past life of Juli's. It had all the signs of a past-life connection between Jana and her daughter, including the pleading phrase, "Please, don't go!"

We investigated the after-death behavior. After he left the body he did not go to the Light. The next experience he could recall was floating through an open window into a house and where he joined Juli. She was four years old.

Dr. B.: "Do you recognize anyone else in the house?"

C.: "Yes. The mother. She is my love."

Jana, the girl's mother in the present life, was "his love" in the previous life. "He" found and joined "her" daughter just to be near her. The attachment had nothing to do with Juli in a past life. And Juli had nothing to do with Jana in that past life either.

In the experience of saying good night at home and good-bye at school, this lonely soul was reminded again and again of his feelings of sadness and overwhelming loss he suffered when she left his side so long ago in the meadow, and at the time of his death. This was not Juli's past-life memory but the continuing pain of an attached discarnate entity. The irritating behavior was imposed on little Juli by this Earthbound spirit.

This entity was guilty of nothing but love. He had interfered with the behavior of the child, Juli, for eight years simply to be close to the woman he had loved in another lifetime. He had no difficulty understanding this inappropriate connection. He expressed his love, released from Juli, and moved into the Light.

A few months later Jana called and reported that after the release of the spirit of this man who loved her mother, Juli had not exhibited the clinging behavior again. It was not just diminished; it was totally absent.

Couples Counseling

Couples counseling cannot be complete without a search for attached discarnates. Couples often came to us following a lecture on SRT. For some, releasement sessions seem like the last resort. We feel it should be the first step in relationship counseling.

Grandma and Grandpa

Maria and Talbot had been married ten years. There were no children. They were a happy young couple, comfortable in their relationship. Maria had shiny, jet-black hair and lovely almond-shaped eyes. Her soft, Latin beauty was appealing, and Talbot adored her.

Talbot was a college graduate with growing success in his career. A gentle man, slim, with curly, pale blond hair, he wore glasses and was only an inch or so taller than Maria. She was devoted to him.

Then Maria met Brian, a Vietnam veteran. He was a rough-and-tumble sort of guy, with a scruffy beard and long, unkempt hair. She was enormously attracted to him and felt compelled to be with him. These feelings surprised her. Nonetheless she had to be with him, and would leave Talbot behind and spend several days at a time with Brian.

Talbot was hurt and confused by his sweet wife's unexpected behavior. He tried to be patient and forgiving when she begged to return home to him. She loved her husband, and he loved her. There was no doubt of this.

After a few weeks at home with Talbot, Maria would again feel compelled to be with Brian. It was terribly confusing to Maria, and it was agonizing for Talbot. Brian was not a rogue, but he certainly enjoyed the action.

The couple had been in counseling for some months without success. This situation was very upsetting for both. Maria grew increasingly confused and distraught. Talbot was nearly at the end of his patience and tolerance. Almost in desperation, they decided to try past-life therapy and spirit releasement therapy.

Maria worked well in the altered state. I guided her to locate the source of the present situation. Almost immediately, a voice emerged that adamantly stated it was not Maria.

C.: "I am most certainly involved in the present situation. Who are you and what do you want?"

Maria was surprised at this other "personality" speaking through her, but remained in the relaxed state and allowed the voice to continue. Maria was definitely not a person with multiple personalities. This was something else. I proceeded with the questions.

Dr. B.: "Who are you and what are you doing here?"

C.: "I have a perfect right to be here. I'm her grandmother."

This was clear to me but a startling revelation for Maria. Her grandmother had died when Maria was a child. After some questioning, enough information was revealed and Maria was satisfied that it was the spirit of her grandmother who had attached to her when very young.

Maria was then directed to visualize Brian, her paramour. After receiving permission from Maria's Higher Self to proceed with the remote releasement, the questioning was directed toward Brian.

Another entity emerged and spoke through Maria's voice.

C.: "Why are you bothering me? This is none of your business."

The client requests assistance from the therapist, and this establishes the therapist's right to intervene. Entities resent interference with the status quo and selfishly demand to be left alone. They like things the way they are.

The next question was directed to the grandmother.

Dr. B.: "Do you recognize this entity with Brian?"

C.: "Yes," she replied without hesitation, "It's my husband."

Equally startling, this fact made the situation clear. Her grandfather had died some months before Maria's birth and had found

Brian. It was Grandma and Grandpa who were getting together through the healthy young bodies of Maria and Brian. This situation called for remote spirit releasement.

Apparently, spirits can perceive future events, because somehow the grandfather knew that Maria, who was not even born yet, and Brian, a kid who lived a few miles across town, would someday meet. The grandfather joined Brian and waited. After her death, the grandmother joined Maria, then waited. In the present situation, they had to wait no longer. The grandmother exerted a strong influence on Maria, who assumed the feelings for Brian were her own and followed the compulsion to be with him.

If the grandfather had foreseen or predicted more clearly, he might have joined Talbot and the problem would not have existed. It is also possible that one future choice for little Maria was marriage with Brian. Many alternate future realities are available, depending on the choices that are made along the way. Either the grandfather made an error in predicting the future or he simply chose the wrong possible alternative.

Maria's grandmother and grandfather agreed to release from these two people and go to the Light together, united again in a way that would bring no further harm to anyone. If both agreed, they could reincarnate again and find each other in another lifetime. And Maria, Talbot, and Brian could get on with their lives.

After this session, Maria and Talbot entered couples counseling with a traditional therapist. Maria saw Brian again briefly; the relationship soon ended as the compulsion was gone. About a year after this session, Talbot reported that he and Maria were doing fine in their marriage.

Tom and Jauwi

Val and Tom, a middle-aged couple, were having trouble in their marriage. He was an alcoholic, and this was causing problems for them both. His attitude grew more childish as he aged. Tom had done some past-life therapy and had discovered a past life during World War II. However, that lifetime overlapped his present life, usually a sign of an attached entity. Val was attending a training class in SRT and elected to do a remote spirit releasement on him as a demonstration for the class.

Tom's libido suddenly had begun to diminish three and a half years earlier, and Val had grown impatient with him. Vacationing in Maui at that time, they had visited a cemetery where Japanese residents had been interred after being tortured and killed following the attack on Pearl Harbor.

Jauwi had been a seven-year-old boy who was hiding with his parents and several others. Though born on Maui, they were of Japanese descent. The fear and prejudice of other residents erupted in a killing rage. This family was a target. Jauwi and his parents were discovered and killed by the mob. Jauwi described the pain as his tongue was pulled out and cut off. I moved him quickly forward, out of his body after death, and he watched from there. He could see only a green mist, until Tom walked through the cemetery. The boy was somehow drawn to this big, kind American, and Jauwi entered him. He felt safe there. The presence of this seven-year-old boy had affected Tom's sexual desire since that time.

As Jauwi focused upward, he saw his parents, who had gone into the Light. He happily took their hands, and in a tearful and loving reunion, he also moved into the Light. In the months to come, Tom regained his former vigor and the physical union between him and Val was restored. There was more work to do on his alcoholism, but this session was a major step in saving their marriage.

Ralph and the Roman Warrior

Ralph and Millie had been married over thirty years. After his second heart attack, their relationship began to deteriorate. In session, as they described the relationship and heart attack, Ralph began to feel tingling sensations in his arms. The linguistic bridge induction usually works with such physical sensations.

"If that tingling had words, what would they be?"

"If that tingling could speak, what would it say, right now?"

He could not get any words or communication from the sensations. Nothing. Millie, sitting beside him, seemed to sense the words and was able to bring through the entity's communication. This was remote spirit releasement with the two people sitting right together. It worked.

During the time Ralph had been in the emergency room following his heart attack, an accident victim was brought in. He was dead on arrival, but his spirit was following the body. The spirit moved from person to person in the ER, looking for another body for his personal use. A past-life personality within Ralph's consciousness recognized this spirit as a fellow warrior in Roman times and invited him in. This entity did not like Millie and was creating discord between them. He willingly departed into the Light. The couple remained together.

The case of Ralph and Millie seems to indicate that past-life characters or personalities are still intact within the subconscious mind. They are sometimes dormant, sometimes awake and aware of present circumstances. They can impact the life of the primary personality with annoying and destructive behavior. This is unusual certainly, but it is sometimes encountered in clinical practice.

The Therapist with Firm Boundaries

Carol was a fifty-five-year-old therapist who was interested in metaphysics and the spiritual teachings. She attended a course on channeling. The homework after the first class was to meditate. During meditation she was to open herself up to channel someone who would be for her own highest good. This was the only instruction. In meditation, a spirit joined her and would not leave. She developed a severe pain in her stomach.

In Carol's session, the therapist focused the questions on the pain in the stomach.

Dr. B.: "If that pain in the stomach could talk, what is the first thing it would say?"

C.: "I'm her mother. Don't send me away."

This was a surprise to Carol. Her mother had died of stomach cancer several years earlier.

Dr. B.: "What happened?"

C.: "I've been wanting to join my daughter ever since I died but she's too strong. When she asked for someone for her own highest good to come in, naturally I came in."

Mother's good intentions, coupled with Carol's invitation without discernment, had caused this attachment. Mother's presence explained the pain Carol experienced in her stomach.

With little communication between them, they were ready to separate from one another for this time. Carol discontinued her channeling class. Her stomach pain disappeared.

Unlike true mediumship, in which the controlling spirit leaves after the purpose is fulfilled, the Earthbound spirit who attaches at this invitation may not want to leave. This process is similar to using the Ouija board, except the whole body and mind serve as the divining instrument.

The VA Nurse

Kara worked in a metaphysical bookstore. She had not been in a meaningful relationship for some years. Trained as a nurse, she had worked for years in a Veterans Administration hospital. Like many nurses, she left the work because of burnout. While still at the hospital, she had fallen in love with Trevor, a Marine medic wounded in Vietnam.

On patrol with four other guys, Trevor had been fifth in line as they moved along a narrow dirt road through the jungle. Suddenly there were explosions in front of him. The point man was blown to bits. "Not enough to pick up," as Trevor described it. The second man had half his body blown away. The third and fourth men in line were killed instantly.

Trevor called in the medevac helicopters. Though seriously wounded himself, he picked up the remains of the second man and hoisted him onto the chopper when it arrived. Trevor's lieutenant was aboard and began yelling at Trevor, blaming him for the disaster. Trevor swung his fist at the officer, knocking him cold. Trevor passed out at the same time and remained unconscious for three days. During this period he was transported to the States and placed in the Veterans Administration hospital where Kara worked. He awoke in the hospital. The spirits of his four buddies had joined him.

After Trevor was released from the hospital, he and Kara dated briefly. Trevor was a violent man, and she soon ended the relationship. He went to live in a forest, camping out alone. He continued to suffer serious depression and he eventually took his life. He joined Kara, the woman he loved, as an attached entity. Since that time, she had avoided relationships with men.

In the session, Trevor emerged immediately. He professed love for Kara, and was quite possessive. He refused to leave. As he explored inside himself, he recognized his four close buddies who were killed on the patrol. Each of them discovered attached entities from the time of the Vietnam War and also from their childhood.

Rick was one of the men killed. One of the entities with him was one of his dad's friends who had died in a hunting accident. When he was a young teen, Rick accompanied his dad and the friend. The man stumbled over his own shotgun. It discharged, killing him instantly.

Another of Trevor's buddies was Sam, an African-American. He discovered Min Van Thieu, a teenage prostitute he had known in Vietnam. She died when a bomb fell on the building where she lived. Another entity within Sam claimed to be a member of the Ku Klux Klan. When Sam was nine years old, living in a shack in Alabama with his parents, three Klansmen came to the house, threatened to rape his mama and burn the house. Sam's daddy pulled out a shotgun and blew the head off one of the white racists. Sam was in shock at the sight of this, and the spirit of the Klansman found the young black easily accessible.

The white man hated Sam. Sam hated this racist who had threatened his family many years before. The white man was directed to locate the source of his prejudice, his hatred. Only a few moments passed, and he began describing a former life as a black youth. The slave master had whipped the boy's parents unmercifully. The young black could barely contain his hatred.

Again, the Klansman was directed to another lifetime that contributed to his hatred. He discovered a life as a black slave, this time as a nubile young woman taken from her husband in Africa, brought to America with the express purpose of being a sex slave for a white landowner. She refused to perform the desired acts, and her tongue was cut out. She fervently hated white people.

After he recalled these experiences, I asked this white racist how he felt about Sam, the black man. His reply was immediate.

"I don't hate him; he's a brother."

Sam expressed his feelings about this man who had threatened to rape his mama and burn his house.

"I don't hate him; he's my brother."

The hatred of lifetimes had been healed for these two souls. The entities were glad to move into the Light together.

Further, there were Vietcong clad in black pajamas, women, a baby, Sam's old dog, and slimy dark sludge that was the energy of hatred and prejudice generated in his life as a black. There was also deep resentment and confusion about the war. All these entities lifted to the Light, and the sludge was cleansed. The narratives of all these people had come through Kara's own voice. She was exhausted and exhilarated at the end of the session.

Trevor thought he had let his buddies down. He was the medic and he could not save them and was plagued by survivor guilt feelings. In this session, he had assisted them in lifting their emotional burdens and releasing the entities trapped within each. All had found their way to the Light. Trevor finally understood his service to them. He helped them go home. This erased the guilt feelings carried so long. He was free. He and Kara exchanged their last words of love and he lifted into the Light.

Within three months, Kara met a man, a customer at the bookstore. She felt a spark of interest, the first in a long time. It developed into a lasting relationship for Kara. There was no longer any external influence keeping her from experiencing a loving relationship.

Twin Flames

Judith recalled a past life in Roman times when her husband, an army commander, went into a battle and never returned. She still felt angry about that abandonment in the present life. During the session it was discovered that each of them knew he would not return, yet neither voiced that knowledge. This undelivered communication still caused pain.

As she went into the session, she was bidding him farewell in front of their home. They were of the patrician class, well-off financially. As he walked away, her heart was heavy with grief. A short time later she received word of his death. Anger at him and at the war along with grief and sadness over the loss welled up in her. Their relationship had been passionate; they had been deeply committed. She suffered great loneliness.

She lived a long life, and came into political power in her later years. The intractable anger and sadness remained. After her death, she, as spirit, was directed back to the day her husband left for battle. She watched him bid farewell to his wife. She followed as he walked with heavy steps toward his fate. She saw him slump against a wall sobbing with grief at what he was losing at home and what he knew was coming in the battle ahead. She watched as he spent the long night contemplating what the battle stood for. She did not yet understand the far-reaching significance of this encounter with the enemy warrior and his troops.

She followed him as he rode into the battle, seeing clearly the opposing forces riding toward his men. She watched as the two leaders approached each other, weapons ready. She puzzled over the commander's hesitation to swing his sword in a death blow to the head of the enemy chief. She refused to watch as the warrior's mace began the swing that would, in moments, crush the skull of the commander. She cried out. Her husband, her beloved, was dead and she could not understand his hesitation.

Again, in spirit, she was directed to the moment of their parting in front of their home. This time she was directed to step into her husband's body, come into his mind, look through his eyes, think his thoughts, feel his feelings, and speak as him. She now understood his foreboding and foreknowledge of the outcome of the impending battle. She knew his sadness as he left her, feeling the powerful and overriding emotion and motivation to bring this drama to completion. She still did not know what it was.

As he spent the long night in contemplation, the story unfolded and she began to understand. Three hundred years earlier, two similar men had met on a battlefield in the very region where this battle was to take place. These men were the ancestors of the enemy chief and her husband, the commander. Many of the troops of each army were family members of these two leaders, also descended from the first two opponents. The commander's ancestors emerged the victors in that original battle.

Many family members of both sides were killed that fateful day. Those of the losing army gathered together and raised their voices in a curse on the victors, their families, and their offspring for all succeeding generations. This hatred and vengeance opened the way for dark forces to infiltrate the losing army. The blood lust and arrogance of the victors allowed dark force infiltration of the soldiers of the winning army. This allowed fertile soil for the curse to take root and flourish. This situation called for a posthumous remote releasement for the soldiers in the field and for their progeny. The dark force entities, the dark networks, and the curse had to be removed.

Through the centuries, each leader from his deathbed had passed on to his son the commission to carry on this blood feud. Through many decades, skirmishes had erupted between the two armies. Many men had died through the centuries. Few people knew the origins of the vendetta. The commander had vowed to end this blood feud; he knew only one way to accomplish it.

The commander's wife, as a spirit, watched through his eyes as the battle commenced in early morning. The armies stood motionless at opposite sides of the field. Suddenly both leaders bolted forward, weapons held high, their troops riding beside them like waves of death. She felt his strength and his firm resolve as he rode headlong toward the enemy chief. She saw the eyes of the enemy warrior glow a deep orange as he closed on the commander. A quick glance at the troops revealed the same fiery glow in their eyes. Dark force entities were pushing many soldiers into senseless battle and certain death.

At the critical moment, she felt the commander hold back in the death swing of his weapon. The troops could not notice, but she knew that the split second of hesitation sealed the fate of her beloved husband, the commander of these loyal troops. A moment later the heavy, spiked mace crashed through his helmet, pierced his skull, and destroyed his brain. He fell to the ground, dead. She was horrified, yet she finally knew the meaning of his sacrifice.

She scanned back through the past-life paths of the commander and the enemy chief. Each was the reincarnation, twelve times removed, of the leaders of the armies that clashed in the original battle three hundred years before. The curse had been passed, along with the commission to continue the battle, from father to son for generations. The karmic burden of these men and their extended families, reincarnational and genetic, was brought up again this terrible day for either resolution or continuation.

The choice was up to the commander. He had killed his opponent in the first battle. He knew he had to die to balance that karmic debt and halt this continuing downward spiral of death. Only then would the senseless feud end. By hesitating, he had made his choice. It was balanced, but at enormous personal cost to himself and his beloved wife.

Yet it wasn't ended by his noble and spiritually valid decision. The DFEs that had infiltrated these souls over twelve generations opposed karmic justice. The situation required group release of the DFEs and dark networks from the opposing armies, on the day of the commander's death and also of the original battle.

The Rescue Spirits of Light were summoned for this release. Archangel Michael and the Legions of Heaven were called to follow all the threads of the dark networks affecting each soldier. The call was put out for all the Beings of Light necessary for cleanup of this group remote release, which spanned centuries. Judith described the dark ones flowing across the sky toward the Light, so closely packed together, they looked like a river of lava.

The commander rose up from his body. He wasn't ready to go to the Light. His thoughts turned toward home and his wife, and he considered going to find her. This was not a loving thought. He voiced the intention to possess her, claiming ownership; he was still influenced by the DFEs. The Rescue Spirits of Light were called to clear the Roman commander. This was accomplished quickly, and he was ready to go to the Light.

The spirit of the commander's wife separated from him and he lifted fully into the Light. She was directed to return to the moment of her own death, many years after his battlefield death. As she lifted toward the Light, she saw and recognized his spark, bright and clear, awaiting her return. As she moved fully into the Light, her spark joined and blended with his; they became one spark. Twin flames were united once more.

Beyond anything else, more fundamental than any technique or process, the most vital and essential aspect of this clinical paradigm is the infinite and eternal healing power of nonjudgmental, unconditional love.

– 13 –
Remote Spirit Releasement: Long Distance Healing

Remote spirit releasement is done at a distance for another person. In other words, the person needing such assistance is not physically present in my office with me. The client in front of me acts as intermediary, a surrogate, on behalf of the target person, the one who needs the releasement work.

It is essential that the entity or entities attached to the target person not be invited or allowed to incorporate into, attach to, speak through, or control the surrogate, our client, in any way. The surrogate is not required to channel the entities. That would amount to inviting a possession of the person acting as the intermediary. Like a simultaneous translator at the UN, the surrogate relays the words of the entities once the intruders are discovered.

In some cases, the target person requests help with the remote session, or gives permission for our client to act as intermediary for the remote work. Without this express permission we ask for Higher Self permission to go ahead with the remote releasement. We ask the client to visualize or sense the target person as if standing in front of her. Once this is done, either in a visual image through eye-to-eye contact, or feeling the other's energy, we ask the client to sense the response to the following request:

Dr. B.: "I call out for Higher Self permission to proceed with this work on [the target person's name]."

Almost without exception, the client feels a warmth, a pleasant tingling, sees a smile or nod on the face of the target person, or senses an emphatic "yes." This is our permission to proceed. If the answer is "no," we stop the process immediately.

Next the client is guided to declare a safety boundary, a do-not-pass zone, to prevent any attempted attachment by the entities with the target person that we are contacting. She is directed to listen and repeat as we say the words, phrase by phrase.

Dr. B.: "To any and all others, I refuse you permission to control my voice, my body, or my mind in any way. I do not give you permission to come close or to control me in any way. And I will repeat your words."

Occasionally an especially intrusive entity will still attempt to control the body of the intermediary. This will show in the posture and movement, facial expression, or the voice. I demand in the name of the Light that the entity back away, and reiterate the client's refusal of such intrusion. It usually works.

Once the connection is established, Higher Self permission is received, and the safety boundary has been declared, I ask the same discovery questions I would for any SRT session. The client in the office listens and repeats the words of any entity responding to the questions. In remote releasement procedures, the process is the same as direct releasement. The client becomes the connecting link, the communication line to the target person at a distance, and the entities can be discovered and released appropriately.

Results of the remote work are definite and specific. Occasionally there is no discernible change. In most cases, there is change that is obvious to the person who received the remote work and the client who acted as intermediary. We are delighted to hear reports from clients about success in their efforts. It is a loving and courageous gift for the target person.

Rescue Work

Groups of EBs can be released from disaster sites such as plane crashes, volcanoes, landslides, earthquakes, battlefields, sunken ships, and the terrorist attack on the World Trade Center in New York on September 11. Groups of DFEs and dark networks can be released from locations such as the Nazi death camps, battlefields, geographical locations, and countries dominated by malevolent dictators.

This requires a team of people, from two to six or more, some of whom have psychic abilities and can perceive and describe the situations. This is called rescue work, and it has been carried on quietly for decades, perhaps centuries. Since time and distance are meaningless in the spirit reality, rescue work can be accomplished on events from long ago.

My First Remote Spirit Releasement

My first request for remote spirit releasement came in 1982, after I had left my dental practice. The client was in the process of divorcing, yet she still had love for her husband and wanted to help him in this manner. She described the situation: his personality changed when he drank alcohol. This is not uncommon, and she recognized the same personality emerge every time, and suspected an interfering entity.

For the induction, I guided her in the Sealing Light Meditation, and she moved easily into the altered state. I suggested she bring an image of her husband into awareness. The image was cloudy, unclear; she couldn't make a connection. I suggested she focus within herself to search for any attachments. She immediately discovered several, and they were released appropriately.

Again I asked her to bring in an image of her husband, and there was an immediate connection. From this case, I learned to clear the intermediary, in this session, the wife, before proceeding with remote spirit releasement. It seems few people on Earth are clear of attaching entities, and this condition interferes with clear connection to the target person. When the client connected with her husband, I requested and received Higher Self permission to proceed.

I asked the client if she could perceive any shapes or shadows, faces or forms around her husband's body, especially the head and shoulders. She stated that she saw three faces. I focused my intention on the one causing the trouble:

Dr. B.: "I call out to the one in charge. I call to the one who takes over when the man drinks. Step forward and speak out!"

Her face twisted into an expression of anguish and disgust.

C.: "That's the one! That's the one I see when he drinks! He's ugly! That's the one I hate!"

Dr. B.: "You, 'ugly', what's the first thing you would say to us? (Then, in a softer voice to the client) What does he say?"

This one was arrogant, belligerent, and caustic.

C.: "What do you want? Why are you bothering me?"

We were in contact with the entity immediately. This one and the other two were released into the Light. She reported that her husband appeared very peaceful. She was greatly relieved. It was a loving thing she had accomplished for him.

Attached Entities from the Nazi Death Camps

Occasionally we discover an attached entity who recalls dying in one of Hitler's death camps in Nazi Germany. They may be attached to the client who also died there and then reincarnated. Such an entity might be attached to a tourist who walked near the camp. There might be no connection whatsoever.

With remote spirit releasement techniques, we can help to release many of those tortured people who died and remained Earthbound during that dark period. We also find Earthbound souls of German guards who knew what they were doing was wrong, but continued for fear they would be killed if they objected to the hideous atrocities. We conduct this rescue work whenever a camp victim is discovered.

Vietnam and Other Battlegrounds

We have discovered many casualties of the Vietnam War attached to clients of both sexes. One woman of about forty discovered the Earthbound soul of a young soldier who was buried in a cemetery in Bakersfield, California. At age thirteen, she traveled there from Los Angeles to attend a graveside service for her cousin killed in an automobile crash. The young soldier was sad because his mother often visited a cemetery in Minnesota, his home, and placed flowers on a grave there. The military had mixed up the burial. He was buried in the wrong state. Through him we reached remotely to the killing fields of Vietnam and released many EBs of combat casualties, American and "enemy."

We also assist EBs of the casualties of the Vietnam War who hover near the Vietnam Memorial Wall in Washington, D.C. Additionally, many naval officers and enlisted men remain as spirits aboard the battleship *Arizona*, sunk on December 7, 1941, during the attack on Pearl Harbor. It remains a commissioned ship of the U.S. Navy; they are duty bound as well as Earthbound. Many soldiers are still suffering from their wounds on the battlefields of the Civil War.

Such places hold the Earthbound souls of people who died in terrible circumstances, surrounded by the intense emotion of combat. The rescue work frees countless lost souls from around the world.

Earthbound Spirits from Hiroshima

A few years ago, we were invited to Japan as the guest of a renowned healer. He had attended a lecture on SRT at a conference in Atlanta and insisted we come to his homeland. He had never before heard anyone describe the conditions that he found in so many of his clients.

While in the country, we did some rescue work on the victims of Hiroshima. Judith perceived some of the Japanese peasants still walking along the old streets, in and out of bamboo and wooden houses and shops. They died so quickly, they continued as if still alive, creating a thoughtform replica of their neighborhood. Others were spinning through space, carried by the force of the blast. We requested as many beings of Light as necessary to take home as many of these lost souls as possible. In every case of group rescue work, some remain stuck and simply will not leave.

Earthquakes

Shortly after the October 17, 1989, Loma Prieta earthquake in northern California, participants in an SRT training course requested a demonstration of remote spirit releasement and rescue work focused on the casualties of that disaster. Despite extensive destruction in the Bay Area, only sixty-three people lost their lives in the quake.

The woman chosen as the demonstration subject was clear in her visual imagery. Judith and several others in the room also received clear impressions as the demonstration proceeded.

The Sealing Light Meditation was used for the altered state induction and invocation of light. I directed the invitation to those who had lost their lives during and after the quake. The wording of the invitation must be specific.

Dr. B.: "In the name of the Light, I call out to those people who suffered in the earthquake. I call out to you and invite you here to this place. This is a place of safety, this is a place of rescue, a place of peace. We welcome you to this place."

The demonstration subject immediately perceived dozens of spirits moving toward her. One participant sensed a mother with a baby in arms. Apparently, many of the Earthbound souls answering this summons had lost their lives in the earthquake of 1906, more than eighty years earlier. Another participant recognized spirits with Asian features. A few weeks prior to the Loma Prieta temblor, a devastating earthquake in China had taken the lives of thousands.

The subject reported the presence of countless light beings ready to assist this rescue. She laughed as the image of a fire engine suddenly came into her awareness.

C.: "They're even coming to the rescue in a fire engine. The rescue squad of the spirit world. But it's like the Keystone Cops."

The beings of Light have a gentle sense of humor, but they don't do slapstick comedy. This sort of cartoon image or caricature was not consistent with the nature of the higher beings.

Dr. B.: "Look at the eyes of the driver. What do you perceive?"

C.: "Oh! The eyes are red! They aren't here to help at all. They're trying to capture some of the earthquake victims."

Apparently this observation was accurate. The DFEs wanted to muscle in on the group rescue and try to pick up a few stragglers, like hyenas picking off the weak members of a herd. They projected the image of a recognized symbol of hope, the trusted fireman, everyone's friend. Being surreptitious and quiet about their dirty work, they would more easily escape detection. They seem to approach many situations such as this with the same stupidity.

Two years earlier, a large earthquake in Armenia had caused widespread destruction and loss of life. Rescue workers flew in from other countries with supplies to assist. One of the planes carrying rescue workers crashed, killing everyone aboard.

Gina, an Armenian by descent, wanted to do a remote session for these people. Easily entering altered state, she perceived clear images. In spirit, one woman was trying to pull at the rubble in a futile effort to free her husband and son. She could not move even a particle of physical matter. Through Gina, she was urged to focus her gaze upward. Her loved ones were in the Light waiting for her.

As Gina searched the area, she discovered spirits of the rescue workers who had died in the plane crash. They were still trying to help. Many of these lost souls were directed to the Light.

Terrorism

The events of September 11, 2001, left an indelible scar on the fabric of human consciousness across the globe. In the attack on the World Trade Center twin towers in New York City and the Pentagon in our capital, more than three thousand people lost their lives within a few minutes, in the buildings and in the passenger airplanes used as weapons.

There was an outpouring of love, sympathy, and solidarity from people around the world, even those from countries not so friendly with the United States. This was a magnificent show of connectedness of all life.

There was also anger, and a need for vengeance and retribution against the perpetrators of the attack. Attention was focused on those who apparently financed and trained the dead terrorists. The president declared a war on terrorism.

A war of retaliation is a form of "fighting fire with fire." It is the same attitude and mind-set that drive the attackers. It is an attempt to solve the problem at the level of the problem, which may not solve the problem without creating additional problems. It is spiritual work that will bring closure to the explosive issues involved.

Many people who are aware of spirit releasement procedures conducted rescue work for the lost, confused souls of the victims of 9/11. SRT work was also directed toward DFEs who controlled the terrorists, fueled their hate, and urged them to give their lives in such an attack. It was not religious zeal but the insanity of terrorism that drove their evil behavior; the God of their professed religion expressly forbids taking human life.

We receive many reports of success with remote spirit releasement, and trust that the process will have some effect on terrorists. Rescue work for lost human souls following disasters, natural or man-made, has been carried on for centuries.

Posthumous Remote Releasement

Katherine scheduled a session for past-life therapy. She wanted to uncover any past lives that were interfering with her present life. Her twenty-one-year-old daughter, Julie, had died three months earlier in a traffic accident while riding on a motorcycle with her boyfriend. Julie had been living at home and had a two-and-a-half-year-old child. Katherine had adopted her granddaughter, knowing that Julie had not been financially or emotionally capable of caring for the child. Her daughter had always been a problem: unruly, defiant, and generally unpleasant.

The exploration of past lives was significant for Katherine. The process led to the Planning Stage for her present life. She examined the plans for personal interactions with significant other people in her coming life. When she came to Julie, her face contorted, her voice tightened.

C.: "She just came in to irritate me. She just came in to make my life harder. Ooooh, she came to be like a burr under a saddle."

Such planned interaction is often for the benefit of the one who feels like a victim. It can be a spiritual lesson in patience, forgiveness, and a balancing for prior-life injustice. This realization normally prompts the exploration of the connecting lifetimes involved. In her case, this possible avenue was not pursued. Her focus suddenly shifted to a viewpoint above and behind Julie and her boyfriend on the motorcycle just before the fatal accident. It was as if she were riding in a traffic helicopter describing the scene.

C.: "Oh God, I can see them. If there is anything to this possession stuff, there is a big black thing on her back. It's making her tell her boyfriend to pass the truck they are following. He's doing it. Oh my God, there's a car coming. Oh my God, they just crashed!"

Katherine was shaken by this imagery, but she continued the narrative.

C.: "She's floating here with this black thing dug into her back. It's always been with her. I remember watching her one time when she hit her brother. She was sitting down in a chair and I saw her literally propelled out of the chair. She didn't stand up, she just lifted out of the chair and landed on her feet. She ran over to him and hit him. I watched the whole thing. She looked at me afterward with such a pitiful expression on her face. She cried to me that she hadn't done it. Now I know she was right."

Dr. B.: "I call on the Rescue Spirits of Light to surround this black thing in a capsule of light. Remove this thing to its appointed place in the Light. They will be gentle with her, Katherine."

C.: "No they're not. They're ripping it off her and they're racing off in the other direction. Oh, she looks so sad. She's looking at me."

Dr. B.: "I call on the Mercy Band of Rescue Angels from the Light. Here is a lost soul, she needs help."

C.: "There is a man in a white suit. He looks kind. He says he can help her."

This was a true guiding spirit from the Light. Katherine and her daughter Julie spoke with each other and quickly reached a mutual understanding and forgiveness. This was a beautiful healing, long overdue. They completed their communication.

Dr. B.: "Julie, we send you to the Light, with love. Farewell."

Some time after the session, Katherine reported that her adopted child's behavior had suddenly improved. She had been manifesting the "terrible twos." That eased considerably. There was no exploration of the connection of Julie with her daughter, but perhaps there had been some influence. Katherine was much happier in her life.

Posthumous remote releasement seems to have a religious equivalent. Biblical scholars have long puzzled over the following verse:

"Now what of those people who are baptized? What do they hope to accomplish?" (1 Corinthians 15:29)

The baptism ritual includes a minor exorcism. In the Mormon faith, members can be baptized for the dead with the intention of clearing the sins of those who can no longer do it for themselves. It is a presumptuous yet compassionate act. It might be considered an act of posthumous remote spirit releasement.

The Nonlocal Connection

The phenomenon of channeling, or allowing another consciousness to speak through one's voice, is well documented.[1] Remote viewing (perception of a location or activity at a distant place or time) has been studied and verified in careful experiments.[2] The power of prayer to heal at a distance has also been established in a number of studies.[3]

This ability to connect might be described as a psychic gift, though most clients can accomplish a remote connection in altered state. This is described as "nonlocal connection."[4] It can also be considered evidence of universal oneness, a basic spiritual principle defining the connectedness of all things, everywhere and everywhen.[5]

Remote communication may be possible in this manner with beings who are: "backward" or "forward" in time; distant in space;

alive or deceased; apparently in other dimensions, whatever that means. There seem to be no barriers to such remote viewing and remote communication, and therefore, to remote spirit releasement.

Psychiatrist Colin Ross, M.D., describes an unusual case from his practice.[6] The phenomenon could be channeling, past-life connection, multiple personality, or possession. Bill, a middle-aged man, sought counseling for his recurrent dreams of the Middle East. The dreams turned out to be a true and accurate déjà vu. While he was on a vacation in Turkey, his dream took on reality as he found familiar sites and buildings. In an altered state session with Dr. Ross, Bill was able to speak for a young boy, Androkleus, who identified himself, his family, and his location in Didyma, Turkey.

Androkleus could hear Dr. Ross's voice from a point above and behind him and would carry out his requests. Ross asked Androkleus to walk to the temple and engage in conversation with the priests or learned men in that place. The twenty-minute walk to the temple took twenty minutes in real time in Dr. Ross's office. The experience could not be hastened by hypnotic suggestion.

Typically, a memory of an event, in this or a past life, can play over and over with the same repetitive detail. This did not happen with Bill in this session. It seemed to be happening in real time in both locations. In a past-life regression, the character doesn't respond to the therapist as Androkleus did. There is no responsive conversation with other characters as if there were a phone link. Yet it happened in this case.

Charissos, the temple priest, was willing to converse with Dr. Ross through Bill's voice, but wouldn't speculate on exactly what he thought Ross was. Charissos knew of multiple personalities, more than one "person" in one body, but did not have an explanation. He was aware of possession and channeling, such as the oracle at Delphi, yet as he spoke through Bill's voice, he did not proclaim any mystical wisdom or knowledge of the future. This was not a channeled entity seeking to be a guru.

Ross speculated the link was some sort of hole or rift in time and space that connected Bill's mind with the mind of Androkleus. Bill, the client, lost interest in the phenomenon and soon stopped the sessions. Although there were few interactions with Androkleus and Charissos, the mystery opened up more questions than it solved: real time, there and here; active, coherent conversation between persons separated by over two thousand years; A communication link through time/space? Apparently, there is no barrier in altered states of consciousness. It is an altered state of reality.

When a client in an altered state is recalling and reliving an alien abduction experience, there seems to be a nonlocal yet real connection with the event itself. We can use the remote techniques and speak with the ET who performs the physical examination or implantation of the communication/monitoring device. Time as it exists on Earth is not the same for the aliens. The dimension we call time is completely malleable for the ETs.

Although I don't understand this, I have observed the success of the techniques of past-life regression, spirit releasement, and remote spirit releasement. Extrapolating from the success witnessed countless times in sessions, I have come to accept the validity of these distant, nonlocal connections and trust that something beneficial has been accomplished through the remote work with aliens and their civilizations. Intuitively I know the work leads to healing of many souls in those distant places, and perhaps in other dimensions.

In view of the success of the direct spirit releasement and the remote spirit releasement work where the results can be observed and substantiated, I accept the probability that rescue work also leads to the healing of many lost souls.

– 14 –
Who Am I?

Several friends attended a lecture on past-life regression, spirit releasement therapy, and recovery of soul fragmentation. After the lecture, we gathered at our friend Ed's house for snacks and conversation. The subjects presented at the lecture are stimulating, sometimes threatening, and incredible to many. Ed had paid close attention during the entire lecture. Now he seemed lost in thought. He was contemplating the possibilities in his own life, considering his own big picture.

He was manager of a large municipal organization with many employees and widespread operations in the area where we lived. It was his job to understand and manage the "big picture." Ed was deeply serious, even somber as he posed this question: "If all this is true, then who am I?" He had grasped the information in a way few people are willing to do. He was clear that it could, and most likely did, apply to himself, his personality, and his life choices. And he was concerned. I had to search my own experience to formulate a cogent response.

Significant changes in personality, behavior, addiction, and life choices are usually slow to happen through psychoanalysis or traditional talk therapy. However, one session of past-life exploration often changes a lifelong problem such as terror of public speaking, fear of heights, snake or water phobia, even signs and symptoms of physical disease.

A woman who lives as a victim, first of child abuse, later of spousal violence, can change that mental framework, her very ground of being, and the victim role will no longer control her life. A colleague described such a case referred to her by the domestic abuse court. The woman, who had been physically abused as a child, revealed that she knew if she acted in a certain way just one more time, her husband, who never had been a violent or abusive man, would hit her. She smiled as she made this statement. "After, all, it proves he loves me." This is terribly distorted thinking. It was conditioned abnormal behavior from her childhood situation.

This sort of distortion is not uncommon. Exploring past lives will reveal other instances of victim behavior. Locating the connecting event when she was the perpetrator would end this downward spiral of violence, perhaps for future lifetimes as well as this life.

Sexual abuse and suicide are not uncommon in cases of DFE infestation. The dark influence distorts the thinking, provokes the base desires, and encourages destructive behavior toward self and others. In more than twenty years of clinical investigation, we have found few people not bothered to some degree by dark force infestation.

Drug addiction is a death sentence for many addicts. Releasing the tortured soul of a deceased drug addict can free both the entity and the living person. Some marriages are definitely not made in Heaven, but are the result of attached entities influencing the choices of two people to wed. Following release of the intrusive entities, the individuals involved are able to reexamine the available choices.

Releasing an attached entity will often end specific behaviors, such as the woman who discarded half her wardrobe because her deceased mother was attached, influencing her taste in clothing, or the woman who was bulimic for twenty-one years because she followed the entity's suggestions, "Eat, it will make you feel better," and "Throw up, it will make you feel better." For one man whose burning desire to dress as a woman had been a tragedy in his life, the releasement session was a miracle.

Tessa and the Strong Man

Tessa was twenty-something, a vivacious, tall, lean young woman. She worked for a package delivery company that enforced the requirement that their drivers must be able to lift a seventy-pound package. She enjoyed the activity, the freedom of the job, not being confined to a desk. Her mother, a practicing hypnotherapist, completed our basic SRT training course.

Her mother enlisted Tessa to serve as a practice subject. They discovered an attached EB, a man who had died in his prime, a strong, independent fellow. Following the procedures, the entity was released, more than willing to leave the body of the young woman and move into the Light with the prospect of reincarnating again as a man. All well and good; however, Tessa was no longer able to heft the heavier packages. She no longer fulfilled the seventy-pound requirement. End of job.

Ansel Bourne

The case of Ansel Bourne, a man who experienced a total change of personality and life circumstances in the beginning months of 1887, was described by William James.

Rev. Ansel Bourne of Greene, Rhode Island, was by trade a carpenter. Following temporary loss of sight and hearing under very peculiar circumstances, he became converted from atheism to Christianity just before his thirtieth birthday. He lived, for the most part, the life of an itinerant preacher for twenty years. Following the death of his first wife, he soon married a widow who insisted he remain closer to home. He resumed his carpenter's trade.

Subject to headaches and periods of depression, he experienced a few episodes of unconsciousness lasting an hour or less. Aside from an area of decreased sensitivity on his left thigh, he was in good health with good strength and endurance. In his community he enjoyed a reputation of firm self-reliance and uprightness of character.

On the morning of January 17, 1887, Bourne drew $551 from his bank in Providence, paid for a certain plot of land in Greene, paid some bills, and got into a Pawtucket horse-car. It was the last thing he remembered. Nothing was heard or seen of him for two months. Police sought in vain to learn his whereabouts.

On the morning of March 14 at Norristown, Pennsylvania, a man calling himself A. J. Brown, who had rented a small shop six weeks earlier and stocked it with stationery, confectionery, fruit, and small articles, and quietly plied his trade, woke up in a fright. He called the people of the house and asked them where he was. He said his name was Ansel Bourne, that he was entirely ignorant of Norristown, and knew nothing of shopkeeping. The last thing he remembered—as if it were yesterday—was drawing out money in Providence and getting into the horse-car.

During the six weeks as A. J. Brown, he had not seemed eccentric or unnatural to anyone. Now they thought him insane, and telegraphed Providence. His nephew came to set things straight in Norristown and to take him home. He was so horrified by the idea of a candy store that he refused to step foot in it again. He had no memory of the episode and found he had lost twenty pounds during the period.

In June 1890, Dr. James conducted hypnotic sessions with Bourne. In trance, the Bourne personality disappeared, and A. J. Brown spoke clearly of his two month episode in Norristown. He claimed he had only heard of Ansel Bourne, had never met him, and did not know Bourne's wife. There seemed no motive for the wandering except there was "trouble back here," and he "wanted rest." In the altered state trance, he looked old, the corners of his mouth turned down, his voice was slow and weak, and he tried vainly to recall time before and after the Norristown episode.

James had hoped to integrate the personalities, to make the memories contiguous, but this did not happen, "and Mr. Bourne's skull to-day still covers two distinct personal selves." He said the case apparently should be classed as one of spontaneous hypnotic trance, persisting for two months. Nothing of the sort ever occurred in the man's life. In most similar cases, the episodes recur and produce significant changes in the person's conduct.[1]

James's reference to "two distinct personal selves" indicates an attached entity, though James does not verbalize such a suggestion. His interest in spirit possession and multiple personality was developing at the time.

Max and Duane

Walter Young described a case of ostensible adult onset of multiple personality disorder, now termed dissociative identity disorder. Duane, a veteran of World War II, began having dissociative episodes after being discharged from the navy. Duane did not drink or use drugs. He described an inner voice that had been present since the war that sometimes advised suicide.

Duane had lived an unhappy childhood, but there were not the usual precipitating factors leading to MPD. Duane and a friend named Max had joined the navy together. In a tragic episode, Duane ordered Max to stand Duane's gunnery watch. A Japanese plane strafed the area and Max was fatally wounded. Duane was with Max in the last moments and heard Max promise, "I'll never leave you." Duane felt responsible for the death of his friend.

With Duane under hypnosis, "Max" claimed to have entered Duane because Max held Duane responsible for his death. He claimed that he had a score to settle with Duane because, "It wasn't my time to die." He denied the presence of any other alters. He acknowledged that he was the "voice" that Duane heard. He took full control occasionally, and Duane was amnesic during these periods. Max lived a hedonistic lifestyle when he was in control of Duane's body, which included riding motorcycles, sexual promiscuity with women, and successfully urging Duane to leave home on repeated trips.

Previous psychiatric records revealed that a dissociative condition was suspected. Max revealed that the former psychiatrist knew of his presence and had attempted to "banish" him. He just went away briefly and returned after the psychiatrist was gone. This is the result of inadequate knowledge of the spirit releasement process.

Duane left therapy with Dr. Young after three months. His anxiety increased as hypnotic sessions were pursued with the intention of exploring the war and early life experiences.

In the discussion, Dr. Young suggests several unusual aspects of the case. Adult onset of MPD is little studied, poorly understood, and considered rare. A single alter in a case of MPD is highly unusual. His discussion attempted to explain the case in psychoanalytic terms but held no concrete conclusions.

The description of the case of Duane and Max is typical of spirit attachment. There are many specific indications, including the following:

1. There was no history that would indicate the antecedents of MPD.

2. The two were friends.

3. Duane was present at the time of Max's death.

4. Duane felt guilt, Max felt blame, an exact fit of emotions.

5. Max promised, "I'll never leave you."

6. Max stated that he had entered Duane, a clear description that the therapist must accept as valid.

7. The voice urged suicide as a way of assuaging blame and guilt and achieving peace for both. This is typical of the influence of the DFEs exacerbating feelings of revenge in a human mind. The idea of achieving peace is a manipulative deception.

8. With Max in control, Duane was amnesic of the lifestyle adopted by Max. This is a case of occasional complete takeover.

9. Max knew he was a separate being and resisted the former psychiatrist's efforts to banish him. Max was not confused by the situation.

10. The situation worsened with further inadequate and inappropriate treatment. Psychiatric intervention was obviously the wrong treatment approach for the condition.[2]

Who Committed the Crime?

The inmates at the women's prison where I volunteered briefly were familiar with entities and discarnate interference. They knew about the "candy striper," a young woman who volunteered at the facility. Candy stripers often help at hospitals, distributing magazines, candy, and such. This volunteer, however, was not alive in her own body, but was an entity, or ghost, as the inmates described her, which roamed the rooms and corridors of the center. Several inmates, and the supervisor who was in attendance at my lecture, claimed they had seen the apparition.

One inmate asked an interesting question: "Can they ever leave once they attach?" I knew she must have good reason to ask such a question.

"Sometimes they seem to be able to leave. Why do you ask?"

"I shot a clerk in a convenience store. I don't know how I got there. Suddenly I was standing over him holding a gun and he was lying on the floor bleeding. I think someone else shot him and then left me. That's why I'm in here."

It would have been a fascinating session if we could have arranged it. If we had confirmed her suspicions in the session, it would have been my second case in which the entity that orchestrated a shooting had exited following the crime, leaving the living human to take responsibility.

In the earlier case, a woman wanted to explore a specific situation she had read about in the news. A man had been executed for shooting a psychiatrist. He swore he was innocent; he had no association with the victim. She did not know the man, but she believed him. In an altered state, she was able to connect with the executed man remotely; the entity who had been with him was also contacted remotely.

The entity was a young man whose mother had been treated by the psychiatrist for schizophrenia. The man had been six years old when his mother was admitted to a mental hospital, from which she was never released. The boy always blamed the psychiatrist for the loss of his mother. He died as a young adult, and attached to another man who had no connection whatsoever to the situation.

In complete control, the spirit of the young man procured a gun, went to the psychiatrist's office, shot him, and separated from the befuddled man who would later stand trial, be judged guilty of the crime, and be executed. It took some explanation before the two men understood the situation and forgiveness could bring resolution. Both lost souls were guided to the Light.

So Who Am I?

In view of these and many similar cases from my practice, and related to me by other therapists, my friend Ed's question, "Who am I?" is profound and far-reaching. Can it be answered? I don't think so. We are all influenced by the values of our parents, schooling, the political climate and current psychological attitudes—in short, the Zeitgeist of the culture.

People who grew up during the Depression in this country have a different attitude toward money than the present generation of young adults who live in a robust economy. They have developed a different attitude about money. All these influences and imprints on our personality are understandable and easily traceable.

Not so obvious are the unseen influences, the spirit factors described in this book. These can be discovered and treated in altered states of consciousness. Unfortunately, many people do not accept the existence of these energies, or the possibility of such energies influencing their minds. This is the present state of knowledge and the prevailing attitude toward such phenomena.

The ideas of reincarnation and past-life memories, spirit possession by discarnate conscious beings, and loss of soul essence lie beyond accepted rational thinking. This is certainly true within the mental health and the medical professions. Yet traditional psychiatry and use of mind-controlling drugs, psychotherapy, and medical treatments are ineffectual in the face of spiritual influences, and humans continue to be affected by all three conditions.

Seeking wider acceptance by the mainstream Western, materialistic, scientifically oriented society, the Catholic Church has increasingly sought to downplay the existence of spirit or demon possession. Cases of distraught people who think themselves possessed are referred to psychiatrists. Except in relatively few instances, the Church fathers have mostly abnegated their responsibility for the spiritual health of people.

However, in the last two decades, this has changed. Some time ago, the Vatican publicly advertised the need for forty exorcists, since so many people in that area were showing signs of possession after involvement in satanic cult activity. Recently a new exorcist was appointed in the Chicago diocese. This event made for sensational news across the country. The present Pope himself is credited with performing three exorcisms since assuming the office.

Within this century, many well-educated, responsible people have investigated the phenomenon of spirit possession intelligently and with purpose. A few have sought an alternative approach to healing the condition. Fortunately, there is a growing number of people who are exploring these unconventional treatment methods for these specific conditions because they work.

And so, Ed, my friend, your question remains an intriguing and unanswerable part of the mystery of consciousness.

Epilogue

Let's take a deeper look at this model of psychospiritual therapy. We can look between the cracks and behind the scenes, as it were. The scientific, metaphysical, and spiritual realities begin to merge, or at least overlap, in the montage of human consciousness.

Past-Life Therapy

Past-life therapy has been a hot topic in the last several decades. Since the controversy sparked by the 1955 publication of *The Search for Bridey Murphy*, numerous books have been written on the subject, many by mental health professionals who use the techniques of PLT in private practice. There is a professional organization dedicated to the study of PLT, which holds annual conferences and offers training courses in the techniques of past-life therapy.[1]

Psychiatrist Brian Weiss produced several books on past-life therapy based on his clinical experience with clients, and has been a prominent figure on TV talk shows. Many people have been introduced to the notion of past-life therapy through his willingness to speak publicly on the use of reincarnation memories in effectively treating patients.

In lectures on the subject, Dr. Weiss has stated that psychiatrists and psychotherapists across the country have called to say they have discovered similar results with the techniques of PLT. Conducted behind closed doors, of course. Most, but not all, mental health professionals consider such memories to be fantasy. Since reincarnation can't exist, then it doesn't exist; *ipso facto*, such memories are fantasy.

Some religious groups have railed against people who speak openly about reincarnation and karma. Though 80 percent of the world's religious philosophies describe some form of reincarnation or reembodiment, and nearly 25 percent of Americans believe in the concept,[2] most contemporary Western religious doctrines exclude any mention of the subject.

John Locke, seventeenth-century English philosopher, regarded the mind of a newborn as a *tabula rasa*, a blank slate upon which experience imprints knowledge. He also believed that all persons are born good, independent, and equal.[3] The notion of *tabula rasa* is contradicted by research in hypnosis and hypnotherapy.

The subconscious and unconscious mind can reveal accurate personal information while a person is in a hypnotic state; this is information that is not retrievable in the normal, awake state. In the altered state, a person can recall details of surgery under anesthesia, early childhood experience, prebirth memories, even events that occurred prior to conception, all of which can be confirmed by parents and others who were there.

When directed to recall earlier events, many people can describe scenes and experiences that seem to be in other time settings, in geographical locations other than their present home, and the person will describe the experience as personal and definitely his or her own.

The magnificent accomplishments of Leonardo da Vinci, Michelangelo, Mozart, Albert Schweitzer, and other such luminaries cannot be adequately explained by inborn talent. It may be possible that we bring with us the skills and abilities from former times, other lifetimes during which we learned and excelled in such pursuits as art, music, healing, mathematics, and statesmanship. Many people who are curious about the purpose and direction of the present life uncover past-life experiences that directly influence and enhance their present-life career, interests, and accomplishments.

Does this prove that reincarnation is real? It is a good indication, not proof. The evidence is empirical, not measurable in scientific terms. There are investigators working on such issues. Dr. Ian Stevenson, Carlson Professor of Psychiatry and director of the Division of Parapsychology, Department of Behavioral Medicine and Psychiatry at the University of Virginia School of Medicine, has made a study of children who remember past lives. These cases come from Burma, Thailand, India, Lebanon, Turkey, Sri Lanka, and the United States.[4]

Stevenson has found that the location of some birthmarks and birth defects seem to be coincident with a mortal wound in a previous lifetime. One well-documented case is Ma Khin Mar Htoo, born in Burma in 1967 with her right leg absent a few inches below the knee. She remembered well her immediate past life when she and her mother walked along the train tracks at Tatkon train station selling flowers. A switch failed to function properly, and a train hit Kalamagyi, her nickname in the former life, while she was walking on the train track and she was killed, her right leg severed a few inches below the knee.[5]

The etheric body memory pattern of a fatal injury can accompany the soul into a subsequent embodiment, manifesting as an illness or physical symptom. Medical intervention may be able to alleviate or eliminate the symptoms, yet the memory pattern that created the condition is still present and may bring about the same condition again. It may also erupt in some other form. These memory patterns can be eased or eliminated through past-life therapy.

Headaches often diminish or cease altogether through past-life therapy. Migraine headaches are severe and recurrent, usually with throbbing on one side, accompanied by nausea and sometimes impaired vision. Cluster headaches are similar to migraines but are of short duration and occur daily over weeks or months, predominantly around one eye. Tension headaches are without consistent location and are thought to result from contractions of the face, scalp, or neck muscles. Guiding a client to the origin or cause of the headaches usually uncovers an event that culminates in the head being crushed by an object such as a rock or tree, or split by a sword or battle axe.

During a lecture, psychologist Dr. Edith Fiore described a case from her files. She met a woman at a social gathering. During their conversation, the woman revealed she was in town for her twelfth or thirteenth bone marrow transplant, part of the treatment for her condition of leukemia. Her sister was to be the donor. The treatment is expensive and painful, and she was not looking forward to the procedure. Dr. Fiore suggested a past-life regression to seek the cause of the condition. The woman agreed. In the session, she discovered herself as the priestess of a religious cult that carried out human sacrifice as part of its ritual. As the priestess, she drank the blood of the sacrificial victim.

The condition of leukemia leads to unrestrained proliferation of white blood cells, usually accompanied by anemia, impaired blood clotting, and enlargement of the lymph nodes, liver, and spleen. The white blood cells overcome the red blood cells, as it were, "consuming" them. So this present-life condition seemed to be the karmic balancing of the past-life activity of consuming the blood of the sacrificial victims. A week following the regression, her physician took bone marrow cells from the sternum by means of punch biopsy. On examination, no abnormal cells were found. The woman did not need a bone marrow transplant. Leukemia was not present.

Dick Sutphen, California-based past-life investigator, trainer, and seminar leader, contends that "wisdom erases karma." Wisdom can come through past-life exploration, as well as spiritual guidance, intervention, and inspiration. He suggests that karma is self-testing and self-punishment, that is, self-imposed. There is no great karmic board that judges and passes sentence on incarnating souls.

Sutphen describes five categories of karma:

1. Balancing karma. This is the simplest form of cause and effect, "an eye for an eye and a tooth for a tooth." A warrior who gouges someone's eyes out in an earlier lifetime might be born blind in this lifetime.

2. Physical karma. This involves the etheric body that carries the pattern of damage from one lifetime to the next. This soul memory pattern imparts similar damage or symptoms to the body in subsequent incarnation. Cases such as the missing lower leg of Ma Khin Mar Htoo, and the diabetic condition of Pete, the TV producer, are examples of this mechanism.

3. False fear karma. Many people suffer from baseless phobias in this life, such as fear of heights, public speaking, or water.

4. False guilt karma. Self-judgment can lead to conditions such as the woman with leukemia just described.

5. Developed ability and awareness karma. Consider the great artists and musicians of history. These extraordinary talents and abilities may have developed over lifetimes.[6]

The hypothetical model of regression therapy is built on spiritual assumptions that seem to fit with observable human responses to the therapist's questions that stem from spiritual assumptions and results that seem to validate the hypothetical model. This circularity is disturbing to me as an investigator and therapist. Perhaps scientific exploration will contribute to the hypothesis.

Dr. Wilder Penfield was one of the world's foremost neurologists and neurosurgeons at the time of his death in 1976. His career spanned more than forty years. One treatment for epilepsy consists of surgically removing a damaged portion of brain tissue that produces erratic electric discharges and causes seizures. This requires removal of a portion of the skull to expose the brain itself. This can be done with local anesthesia so the patient can remain conscious and able to speak. The brain itself has no sensory nerves so does not feel pain. The neurosurgeon can stimulate areas of the brain tissue with a low-voltage electrical probe in order to localize the specific damaged area of brain tissue responsible for the epileptic seizures. This area is cut away, and ideally, the seizures will no longer occur.

In the case he labeled "M. M.," Penfield electrically stimulated the temporal lobe at various points. M. M. reported flashbacks, brief memory bursts, clear, multisensory, "experiential" memories, as vivid as the original experience. Dr. Penfield had located and stimulated the engram, the memory trace of the experience stored in neuronal connections.

The stimulation of the temporal lobe activates a memory record in a distant part of the brain, apparently through the activity of the hippocampus, a bilateral structure in the higher brain stem, adjacent to the temporal lobe. The function of this structure seems to be to store keys-of-access to memories, that is, the record of the stream of consciousness. The scanning and recall of experiential memory is possible.

Two related brain mechanisms are revealed by stimulation of the interpretive cortex. One is subconscious and automatic as neuronal signals interpret the relationship of the individual to his immediate environment. The signal appears in the conscious mind. This is a sort of early warning system, assessing any situation as friendly and familiar, or frightening and threatening.

The second automatic brain mechanism is capable of retrieving a strip of past experience in complete detail. The interpretation of the present situation is compared with the memory record of the past. The memory may be complete with sights, sounds, smells, tastes; that is, multisensory—and I would add, emotional tone.

Though he didn't discuss it, Penfield described the neurological pathways that explain the process of past-life memory recall and make possible the effective use of past-life therapy to correct the distortions in the engram. In turn, this can alter the mind-body programming that leads to present-life disruptions such as crippling phobias and physical disorders such as diabetes and leukemia.

He did not write about stimulation of past-life memories. He was careful to refrain from introspection and speculation, as this would take him outside the confines of any scientific paradigm, inviting criticism from his peers. But he did speculate on the continuation of consciousness following physical death. He could not, as a scientist, find evidence of mind separate from brain, yet he held to the dualistic hypothesis of two elements: mind and brain.

While many others in his field held to the monistic hypotheses—there is only brain—Penfield discovered that nowhere in brain matter could he stimulate mental activities such as belief or decision making. These are higher mind functions. It seemed clear that he believed in mind separate from the physical apparatus of the brain.

In his preface, he made this statement:

> On the basis of either hypothesis the nature of the mind remains, still, a mystery that science has not solved. But it is, I believe, a mystery that science will solve some day. In that day of understanding, I predict that true prophets will rejoice, for they will discover in the scientist a long-awaited ally in the search for Truth.[7]

In my role as teacher of PLT and SRT, I have had to clarify my own thinking and develop more precise descriptions and terminology for the process as I understand it. As I train others in these techniques, I continue to grow in understanding and clients benefit from my learning.

What is the intent of PLT? To uncover memories of the cause and origin of an unwanted present-life condition. The original event is nearly always in the setting of another time and place or another lifetime. Careful exploration of the original trauma that was misperceived and misinterpreted will bring an awareness of the actual nature of that event *as it was*, without the additional mental baggage of judgments, decisions, assumptions regarding self, others, and the situation, and emotional residue of anger, guilt, or fear. This is not a matter of revising history, rather it is discovering the true history of an event.

What is the expected result? Strong emotions, erroneous judgments, false beliefs, and inappropriate decisions connected with the original event are retained as part of the engram. As this is explored and resolved, the client will begin to feel a peaceful resolution of the causal event. This will bring a similar peaceful resolution in the present time. The presenting problem or conflict is healed.

How is this accomplished? As the client describes the present problem or conflict, emotions begin to emerge; these cause physical sensations. Verbal description is used as a trigger, and repetition of the descriptive phrase, often metaphoric, takes the client to memories of earlier events. I suggest this is a function of the mind as *separate* from the physical structure of the brain.

In this process, a sequence of engrams is stimulated, and the stream of consciousness memories emerge. The client is guided to repeat the descriptive phrase and recall an earlier, similar incident when they felt the same way. Emotions build, sensations intensify, the voice becomes louder, and suddenly the engram of a past-life trauma emerges, often in full color and exquisite detail. Following the resolution of the original event, the client is guided to integrate the new knowledge with the present-life situation.

In many cases, the other person (or persons) involved in the conflict will also feel some degree of resolution.[8] The interactions between the client and others will often be eased or healed without any contact between the therapist and the others involved. This non-local connection is fascinating to observe. The same process operates in remote spirit releasement.

In our training courses, we present these concepts in the following way. Any traumatic event in life triggers the reaction termed the "traumatic event sequence." Multisensory perceptions of each succeeding moment of any event are registered by the conscious mind and recorded in the memory banks of the subconscious. These perceptions are always *misperceptions*. There is a distorted and incomplete perception of the actual circumstances of any situation, whether or not traumatic.

One function of the mind is to interpret incoming data. Interpretation of the details of any event is always colored by one's own emotional and mental filters, which leads to faulty interpretation. The interpretations of misperceptions become *misinterpretations* of the misperceptions.

Inaccurate perceptions and interpretations then lead to inappropriate and incongruent decisions such as: "I'll never trust men again," "I will never be rich again," "I can never speak my truth," "I don't deserve . . ." In similar future events, a person will often make the same decision again. A decision which is declared several times becomes a belief, an unquestioned operating principle in a person's life.

Thus the memory of any experience is always distorted. Not completely false, just distorted. It is the distorted memories in the subconscious mind that further distort similar future experiences. It is not only what happens to a person that remains in the memory banks and has the lasting effect, but the mental, emotional, and physical impact of the event. This is the engram, the psychic memory trace.

The engram holds all perceived details, misperceived details, misinterpretations, and the mental, emotional, and physical residues associated with the event. These are scars on the soul.[9] In trance, Edgar Cayce, the "Sleeping Prophet," counseled that these scars must be removed from the mental and spiritual self.[10]

The mind uses the misinterpretations of the misperceptions of any present event to *assess* the present situation for potential danger, that is, a threat to its own survival, by making a *comparison* of this distorted view of the present situation with the distorted memory of any *earlier similar event* that contained a real or imagined *threat to survival.* Faulty *judgment* of the present threat as compared with past events leads to an inappropriate *re-action* to the present event and the persons involved. The inappropriate reactions can be mental, emotional, or physical.

The presenting problem, the chief complaint of the client is the outward manifestation, the mental, emotional, or physical outworking of these inappropriate re-actions. The metaphoric description of the present-life problem or conflict may be an accurate description of the original traumatic event, stimulated by something in the present-life situation that is similar to the earlier traumatic event or situation.

The present re-action is often a repeated action, similar to the response in the earlier event that overcame the threat to survival, allowing the person to survive. The re-action can be physical in cases of food allergy, asthma, skin eruptions, signs and symptoms of illness. The re-action can be emotional upset, phobia, aversion, or attraction to another person or a geographical location or time period.

The re-action can be manifest as a behavior such as overeating, excessive drinking, aberrant sexuality, or drug addiction. Mental re-action such as racial prejudice, attitude toward the opposite sex, decisions and beliefs about self-worth, abundance, or any other unwarranted judgment or assumption can interfere with a peaceful, productive life.

An example of a re-action is the birth regression session in the dental office described earlier. The re-action was her physical sensation and emotional feeling, verbalized as: "I can't get my breath. I just want to get out of here." Another example is the man with the fear of public speaking, specifically, an aversion to the onlookers are staring at him. In a past life he died just as he gazed at the crowd.

The presenting problem, the client's chief complaint, can be considered a re-action to an earlier traumatic event, most often discovered in a past-life setting. It may have been appropriate in that time, it is almost never effective or appropriate in the present. Past-life therapy guides the client in unraveling the distorted emotional, mental, and physical residue connected to the original event. Awareness and understanding of the actual nature of the original event and forgiveness of the persons involved will bring clarity and peaceful resolution to the past-life event and present-life conflict.

Daniel Schacter, chairman of the Psychology Department at Harvard University and a leading memory expert, has developed a framework that describes basic memory imperfections.[11] The seven fundamental "sins" of memory are: *transience,* forgetting over time; *absent-mindedness,* involving a breakdown between attention and memory, a preoccupation with something else that prevents a memory to be registered in the mind; *blocking,* a thwarted search for a piece of information like a friend's name or a familiar phone number; *misattribution,* assigning a memory to the wrong source, mistaking fantasy for reality, or incorrectly remembering the origin of a bit of information; *suggestibility,* referring to memories that are implanted as a result of leading questions or suggestions when a person is trying to recall details of a past experience; *bias* reflects the powerful influence of beliefs, current knowledge, and point of view on memories of the past; and *persistence,* the repeated recall of disturbing information that comes unbidden into conscious awareness.

Two aspects of faulty memory can affect therapy. *Misattribution,* assigning a memory to the wrong source, a false cause. This leads to false blame, and this perception can last lifetimes. The second is *suggestibility,* referring to memories that are implanted by a therapist as a result of leading questions or suggestions. In a therapy session, great care must be taken to frame the questions as open-ended, without emotion, without suggested or multiple choice answers. The questions: "What happened?" and "What happens next?" offer the least intrusive approach to uncovering memories.

These two potential disruptions of memory are also relevant in the legal system, where a defendant's life may hang on the details of memory furnished by a witness. The attorney's suggestive, even coercive questions intrude on the testimony: "Isn't it true that you . . ."

In some cases, persistent memory flashes will bring a person into therapy, where they will discover a particularly painful past-life memory. Prolonged flashes might come in a dream as with Marian, the TV hostess. Once uncovered, it can be resolved, healed, and will not recur again.

In medicine there are false and arbitrary walls which stand between specialties such as endocrinology, neurology, cardiology, and certainly the soft sciences of psychiatry and psychology. A specialist will often ignore other bodily systems in the course of diagnosing and treating a disease condition. Until Candace Pert at NIH discovered neuropeptides, the body's messenger molecules that exist within the brain and throughout the organs and tissues of the body, there was only speculation on the mechanism of communication within the physical body.

It has now been shown in extensive lab work that the brain sends messages to every part of the body. The mind controls what goes on in the organs. Such expressions as "gut feeling," "heartache," "pain in the neck," "headache," take on new meaning. The human body is an integrated organism, not a group of separately functioning, autonomous systems. There are no walls. And this most certainly includes mind and consciousness. The mind is seen by many as the programmer for the brain, the computer system of the body.

Candace Pert and her partner Michael Ruff collaborated on much of the work at NIH. They proposed a name for the new multidisciplinary field they were helping to develop, "psychoimmunoendocrinology," to include the endocrine system, the source of hormones in the body. The term that triumphed, "psychoneuroimmunology," was coined by Dr. Robert Ader who wrote a book by that name. In any case, it is the mind/brain (psycho, neuro) that controls and modulates the defense function (immunology) of the body.[12]

The mind/body connection is firmly established and largely understood in terms of messenger molecules. Emotional reaction activates the communication system, and the body receives the messages. The interpretive cortex assesses the immediate surroundings for threats to survival, the stream of consciousness seeks earlier similar events when there was a threat to survival successfully met and overcome. The response to the earlier event is repeated, the reaction to the present situation.

This system goes beyond the brain if we consider past-life memories as actual experience in the stream of consciousness They are real memories of earlier events in other times and places, the mind embodied in a different body than the present vehicle. Investigators have authenticated details of past-life memories in many cases. This does not prove reincarnation. Some skeptics opt for the explanation of super ESP, without scientific evidence for such a phenomenon.

Whatever the explanation for ostensible past-life memories, the process of past-life therapy is direct, effective, and substantially more efficient than traditional talk therapy. The arbitrary boundaries on human existence have been pushed back by empirical evidence gained from explorations in human consciousness. Near-death experience studies have shattered the notion that life ends at the cessation of body function. Pre- and perinatal therapy have pushed the earliest frontier back to the moment of conception and beyond. Past-life and between-life exploration allows further investigation of the stream of consciousness.

Jung theorized the notion of the collective unconscious, the connectedness of all life.[13] Philosophers and mystics for centuries have proclaimed we are part of the mind of God and connected, part of the totality, the Oneness.

Perhaps quantum physics will eventually provide some answers. David Deutsch, one of the world's leading theoretical physicists, holds the view that all possible events, all conceivable variations on our lives, must exist. We live not in a single universe, he says, but in a vast and rich "multiverse."[14] Bryce DeWitt was the physicist who first coined the term "many worlds" to describe this perplexing idea. In 1957, Hugh Everett wrote his doctoral dissertation at Princeton on the "many worlds" interpretation of quantum mechanics. Initially, there was a resounding indifference toward Everett's work from the world of physics.

The laws of quantum physics insist that the fundamental constituents of reality, such as protons, electrons, and other subatomic particles, are not hard and indivisible, but behave like waves and particles at the same time. They can appear out of nothing and disappear again. They can travel from point A to point B without passing through the space between. On the quantum scale, objects seem blurred and indistinct. A single particle occupies not just one position, but here, there, and many places simultaneously.

Deutsch states that different times are nothing less than different universes. "The universes we can affect we call the future. Those that can affect us we call the past."[15]

A basic metaphysical concept is simultaneous time: past, present, and future exist in the spacious present; all being, all existence, is now. The only separation between things is one of vibrational frequency. Time is experienced as moving from past to future, an effect of the conscious mind. A client occasionally discovers a "future" life as the source of a present-life problem. Such concepts are difficult to grasp.

This is where physics and metaphysics intertwine. In 1964 Irish physicist John Stewart Bell took a sabbatical from the fast-paced world of high energy physics at CERN, the European accelerator center in Geneva, Switzerland, to explore the byways of quantum physics. His exploration led him to formulate what has become known as Bell's Theorem. Essentially, everything is connected to everything else, without regard to physical distance, time, and space that seem to separate everything. The connection is instant, immediate, and eternal.

Remote healing occurs, remote viewing can be quite accurate, clairvoyance and precognition can be verified, a pair of electrons that separate will act as if they are still in contact, no matter where in the universe they travel. Speed of light does not govern such non-local phenomena. The *facts* of quantum physics have proved Bell's Theorem; it does not rely on quantum *theory*.[16]

Spirit Releasement Therapy

As William James stated so eloquently:

> That the demon-theory will have its innings again is to my
> mind absolutely certain. One has to be "scientific" indeed to
> be blind and ignorant enough to suspect no such possibility.

The earliest treatment of mental disorders was practiced by Stone Age cave dwellers some half million years ago. For certain mental disorders involving severe headaches and convulsive attacks, the shaman, or medicine man, performed a trephination, or removal of a circular piece of the skull. This opening presumably permitted the evil spirit causing the trouble to escape. Primitive skulls reveal healing of the edges of the opening, indicating years of life following the procedure.

Demons and devils were considered commonplace in Babylonia and Assyria. Written accounts of the treatment of illness were deciphered from the cuneiform texts of Assyrian tablets dating from about 2500 B.C. Incantations and prayers to the tribal gods were interspersed with direct challenges to the demons that imposed disease of every description.

Many people have believed that there was a nonphysical existence parallel and coexistent with the physical universe. People considered that world to be filled with spirits. Ancients believed that most sickness was caused by evil spirits. In ancient Egypt, the exorcism was performed by a team: a physician to cure the ailment and a priest to drive out the demon.

Early writings of the Chinese, Egyptians, Hebrews, and Greeks reveal that they believed mental disorders were caused by demons that had taken possession of an individual. In ancient Persia of the sixth century B.C., the religious leader Zoroaster founded the religion that became known as Zoroastrianism. Ahura-Mazda was the God of Light, Ahriman was the master of darkness. Zoroaster, considered the first magician, was also an exorcist who used prayer, ritual, and sprinkling of water to drive out evil spirits. In India, the mother of Buddha was considered a great exorcist. King Solomon was perhaps the most noted of the Jewish exorcists.

In the New Testament, one-fourth of the healings accomplished by Jesus consisted of casting out unclean spirits. He specified more than one type of spirit. The Roman Ritual was developed over a long period of time and continues as the model of exorcism in the Catholic Church. This concept of deliverance is loosely based on the explicit command and example of Jesus to "cast out devils," though clergy to this day fail to differentiate among demons, the minions of Lucifer, the Earthbound spirits of deceased humans, and the possibility of extraterrestrials interfering with living humans.

Hippocrates (460–377 B.C.), the great Greek physician, has been called the father of modern medicine. He denied the possibility of deities or demons as the cause of disease. Further, he insisted that mental disorders stemmed from natural causes and, like other diseases, required rational treatment.

The physician Galen (A.D. 130–200) studied and described the anatomy of the nervous system. Among the causes of mental disorders he listed the following: injuries to the head, alcoholic excess, adolescence, fear, shock, menstrual changes, economic reverses, and disappointment in love. With Galen's death, the contributions of Hippocrates and later Greek and Roman physicians were lost in a resurgence of popular superstition and belief in demons as the source of illness.

In the period of the Middle Ages, A.D. 500 to A.D. 1500, there was a revival of the most ancient superstition and demonology, slightly modified to conform to theological demands. Treatment of mental illness was left largely to the clergy in the belief that it was caused by evil spirits.

Not until the sixteenth century, over twelve hundred years after Galen's death, did another prominent physician, Paracelsus (1490–1541), reject demons as the cause of abnormal behavior. He defied the medical and theological traditions of his time, for which he was hounded and persecuted until his death.

Reason and the scientific method gradually led to the development of modern clinical approaches to mental illness. In the face of this ongoing dissent, demonology lost ground. Even so, the belief in demons remained widespread. Mental illness and demonology—the study of demons and spirit possession—have been inseparably linked through the tortuous course of history.[17]

It is worth noting that the three subjects—hypnosis, spirit possession, and multiple personality disorder—were quite acceptable professionally at the turn of the century, then faded virtually simultaneously into obscurity. With the publishing of the book, *The Three Faces of Eve*, MPD once again came into public awareness in 1957.

Hypnosis was accepted by the American Medical Association in 1958 and the American Psychiatric Association in 1962. Treatment of spirit possession never ceased but continued quietly through the years.

Recovery of Soul Fragmentation

Again in the words of William James: "If there are devils, if there are supernormal powers, it is through the cracked and fragmented self that they enter."

James juxtaposed two disparate concepts, self (soul) fragmentation and spirit possession. Working with thousands of clients, we have recognized the validity of his words.

Recovery of Soul Fragmentation

We developed, in 1990, the clinical techniques of Recovery of Soul Fragmentation and since then have been using and teaching this method of healing. Consistency in client's responses and results of treatment suggest the possibility of a common phenomenon of human consciousness.

RSF and Holistic Healing

The term "holistic" stems from the word "wholeness," meaning completeness, totality of body, mind, and spirit. Fragmentation as the source of illness is an important concept in the indigenous healing traditions. Soul retrieval, the shaman's approach to healing soul loss, has been considered by present-day mental health practitioners to be nothing more than magic and superstition.

Past-life therapy is also considered fantasy. Treatment of ostensible spirit possession is ridiculed as a relic of earlier religious superstition. In counseling practice, recovery of soul fragmentation, past-life therapy, and spirit releasement therapy are complementary techniques. The results cannot be denied.

Clinical psychotherapy is derived from empirical observation and methods developed by trial and error resulting from these observations. Unfortunately, in present theories and approaches to therapy, the ancient concept of soul retrieval has not been accepted.

From a wider perspective, the spiritual reality, it is obvious and clearly essential for healing. Recovery of soul fragmentation is an important addition to the field of holistic healing.

PLT and Holistic Healing

Past-life therapy is used effectively by a small number of mental health professionals living in many countries. Through emotional feelings and body sensations associated with an identified present-life problem, the client is prompted to locate the source or cause of the problem. This leads to discovery of a pain-filled memory in a past life. The client, in the personality of the past-life character, is guided through resolution of the traumatic episode in that lifetime, and finally through the death experience. The lifetime with its emotional burden is laid to rest and the present-life problem is no more.

Emotional problems and attendant conflicts are quickly and effectively resolved through past-life regression therapy, typically in far fewer sessions than with conventional therapy. Many physical ailments are considered psychosomatic, and these conditions may diminish or cease altogether through past-life regression therapy.

If reincarnation is valid, then most problems and conflicts suffered in this life stem from other times and places. Current mental health approaches are working on the tree rather than caring for the forest. Past-life therapy is part of the whole picture, the soul's journey, an essential part of holistic healing.

SRT and Holistic Healing

If we are, as many spiritual teachers assure us, spiritual beings enjoying a brief and temporary journey in a physical body on Earth, then we must attend our spiritual needs, personally for ourselves, and for our brothers and sisters no longer in physical embodiment. We cannot exclude the nonphysical conscious beings who need our help. The techniques of SRT have been developed empirically with much assistance from them.

We cannot see bacteria and other microbes without the aid of a microscope, yet they cause illness and death. When swimming, we can see only what is above the water surface. Only 10 percent of an iceberg shows above the water's surface. Scientists tell us we use much less than 10 percent of our brain. Where is the other 90 percent? What is it doing?

Most of us cannot perceive discarnate entities in our normal conscious state, categorized according to brain wave frequency as beta consciousness. We drop into slower alpha and alpha-theta frequencies when we sleep and dream, into delta when the body is in deepest sleep. In altered state therapy sessions, clients seem to enter the alpha and alpha-theta state and can perceive all manner of non-physical beings. Is it imagination, or an innate ability that most people can access and use in such a state? Perhaps heuristic research will give us the empirical answers to such inquiry, along with new meanings of human experience and relevant personal realizations.[18]

Many hundreds of therapists in this country and around the world are using spirit releasement therapy and depossession techniques to assist people affected by discarnate intruders. My first book, *Spirit Releasement Therapy: A Technique Manual*, in English, has sold, or been donated, to therapists and interested individuals in many countries. Other authors have described their own methods for releasing attached entities of various kinds. The work is expanding worldwide as the need is surfacing and the condition is recognized.

Dr. Carl Wickland chronicled his work in his two books. His conversational approach was practical, methodical, and compassionate. Wickland's methods became the foundation for the techniques I began to develop and eventually named spirit releasement therapy.

Used-book stores are a treasure field for me. In my never-ending search, I found a hardcover copy of Wickland's first book. Inscribed in his own hand inside the front cover were these words:

Truth wears no mask
Bows at no human Shrine
Seeks neither place nor applause
She only asks a hearing.

Sincerely, The Author
Carl A. Wickland M.D.
Los Angeles, Calif.
January 26, 1929

These words still thrill me whenever I take the book from its shelf and read them. It feels as if he were reaching out to me across decades with an invitation to continue the work. I have accepted the invitation. It has become my work.

Appendix A
Dissociative Trance Disorder

The American Psychiatric Association publishes the *Diagnostic and Statistic Manual of Mental Disorders*. The fourth edition came out in 1994 and is abbreviated *DSM*-IV. Draft copies were sent to many mental health professionals for comments and reactions to new categories and revised descriptions. More than any other included category, dissociative trance disorder elicited the most vociferous reaction. As a result, the APA committee included the category in Appendix B: Criteria Sets and Axes Provided for Further Study.

The World Health Organization (WHO) developed the *International Classification of Diseases and Related Health Problems*, Tenth Revision (*ICD*-10). The APA and WHO have correlated code numbers and descriptive terms between *DSM*-IV and *ICD*-10. Dissociative disorder NOS (Not Otherwise Specified) is listed as F44.9 in *ICD*-10, and 300.15 in *DSM*-IV. Example 4 in the following section, which is a verbatim excerpt from *DSM*-IV, is titled "Dissociative Trance Disorder," which includes Possession trance. The condition is well known in many parts of the world, and the wording here is quite similar to that included in the text of *ICD*-10.

Dissociative Trance Disorder

Features

The essential feature is an involuntary state of trance that is not accepted by the person's culture as a normal part of a collective cultural or religious practice and that causes clinically significant distress or functional impairment. This proposed disorder should not be considered in individuals who enter trance or possession states voluntarily and without distress in the context of cultural and religious practices that are broadly accepted by the person's cultural group. Such voluntary and nonpathological states are common and constitute the overwhelming majority of trance and possession trance states encountered cross-culturally. However, some individuals undergoing culturally normative trance or possession trance states may develop symptoms that cause distress or impairment and thus could be considered for this proposed disorder. Specific local instances of dissociative trance disorder show considerable variation cross-culturally with regard to the precise nature of the behaviors performed during the altered state, the presence or absence of dissociative sensory alterations (e.g., blindness), the identity assumed during these states, and the degree of amnesia experienced following the altered state.

In trance, the loss of customary identity is not associated with the appearance of alternate identities, and the actions performed during a trance state are generally not complex (e.g., convulsive movements, falling, running). In possession trance, there is the appearance of one (or several) distinct alternate identities with characteristic behaviors, memories, and attitudes, and the activities performed by the person tend to be more complex (e.g., coherent conversations, characteristic gestures, facial expressions, and specific verbalizations that are culturally established as belonging to a particular possessing agent). Full or partial amnesia is more regularly reported after an episode of possession trance than after an episode of trance (although reports of amnesia after trance are not uncommon). Many individuals with this proposed disorder exhibit features of only one type of trance, but some present with mixed symptomatology or fluctuate between types of trance over time according to local cultural parameters.

Associated Features

Variants of these conditions have been described in nearly every traditional society on every continent. The prevalence appears to decrease with increasing industrialization but remains elevated among traditional ethnic minorities in industrialized societies. There are considerable local variations in age and mode of onset. The course is typically episodic, with variable duration of acute episodes from minutes to hours. It has been reported that during a trance state, individuals may have an increased pain threshold, may consume inedible materials (e.g., glass), and may experience increased muscular strength. The symptoms of a pathological trance may be heightened or reduced in response to environmental cues and the ministrations of others. Presumed possessing agents are usually spiritual in nature (e.g., spirits of the dead, supernatural entities, gods, demons) and are often experienced as making demands or expressing animosity. Individuals with pathological possession trance typically experience a limited number of agents (one to five) in a sequential, not simultaneous, fashion. Complications include suicide attempts, self-mutilation, and accidents. Sudden deaths have been reported as a possible outcome, perhaps due to cardiac arrhythmia.

Differential Diagnosis

According to *DSM*-IV, individuals whose presentation meets these research criteria would be diagnosed as having Dissociative Disorder Not Otherwise Specified.

This diagnosis should not be made if the trance state is judged to be due to the direct physiological effects of a general medical condition (in which case the diagnosis would be Mental Disorder Not Otherwise Specified Due to a General Medical Condition) or a substance (in which case the diagnosis would be Substance-Related Disorder Not Otherwise Specified).

Research criteria for dissociative trance disorder

A. Either (1) or (2):

(1) trance, i.e., temporary marked alteration in the state of consciousness or loss of customary sense of personal identity without replacement by an alternate identity, associated with at least one of the following:

(a) narrowing of awareness of immediate surroundings, or unusually narrow and selective focusing on environmental stimuli

(b) stereotyped behaviors or movements that are experienced as being beyond one's control

(2) possession trance, a single or episodic alteration in the state of consciousness characterized by the replacement of customary sense of personal identity by a new identity. This is attributed to the influence of a spirit, power, deity, or other person, as evidenced by one (or more) of the following:

(a) stereotyped and culturally determined behaviors or movements that are experienced as being controlled by the possessing agent

(b) full or partial amnesia for the event

B. The trance or possession trance state is not accepted as a normal part of a collective cultural or religious practice.

C. The trance or possession trance state causes clinically significant distress or impairment in social, occupational, or other important areas of functioning.

D. The trance or possession trance state does not occur exclusively during the course of a psychotic disorder (including mood disorder with psychotic features and brief psychotic disorder) or dissociative identity disorder and is not due to the direct physiological effects of a substance or a general medical condition.

Reprinted with permission from the *Diagnostic and Statistical Manual of Mental Disorders*, Fourth Edition, copyright 1994 American Psychiatric Association. (pp. 727–729)

The symptoms of the trance state (e.g., hearing or seeing spiritual beings and being controlled or influenced by others) may be confused with the hallucinations and delusions of schizophrenia, mood disorder with psychotic features, or brief psychotic disorder. The trance state may be distinguished by its cultural congruency, its briefer duration, and the absence of the characteristic symptoms of these other disorders.

Individuals with dissociative identity disorder can be distinguished from those with trance and possession symptoms by the fact that those with trance and possession symptoms typically describe external spirits or entities that have entered their bodies and taken over.

This proposed disorder should not be considered in individuals who enter trance or possession states voluntarily and without distress or impairment in the context of cultural and religious practices.

Appendix B
Spiritual Protection
by Rev. Judith A. Baldwin

This chapter is excerpted from the forthcoming book on the subject of spiritual protection reprinted here with permission.

When I am lecturing or teaching, the most frequently asked questions are about how to protect ourselves from interfering entities and destructive energies. In my experience, spiritual protection is a way of life. It is not enough to practice techniques, or to rely on ritual or ceremony. For at the end of these, too often there is still the fear to face. What is needed is a practical means of living in a state of invulnerability, regardless of the unexpected, and in spite of the unknown.

Spiritual protection is like a great cathedral built over time. First we lay in place the keystones of spiritual invulnerability. Then we carefully build the archway to spiritual adeptness. Finally, after much practice, spiritual invulnerability is in place and we are ever aware of it.

To be invulnerable requires that we become spiritually adult, as opposed to remaining spiritually childish. Though this is not a particularly complex task, it can seem demanding, probably because most of us would rather be cared for than to care for ourselves. Fortunately, responsibility for keeping the Spiritual Immune System healthy belongs with oneself, and therefore something can be done about it. In fact being spiritually adult looks a lot like a life well lived.

It may help to think of interfering entities and destructive energies as "spiritual bacteria." One is not upset by the idea that the bacteria which plague the physical body must be controlled by daily hygiene. We neither resist nor hide from this reality, we simply bathe, shampoo, and brush regularly. Why then should we be threatened by the reality that we must also perform spiritual hygiene to keep ourselves from being overcome by opportunistic spiritual bacteria?

Let us look closely at how we see ourselves. When you picture yourself do you see a body? When you think of being safe or protected do you mean keeping the physical body safe? When you worry about your loved ones, are you imagining bodily harm? If "yes" is the answer to these questions, you have spiritual homework to do.

We begin our remedial work in primary spiritual education with this realization. No matter what, even if we are sleeping or standing still, we are never guaranteed that the body will not be injured, or sicken, or die in the next moment. If one of the great oaks that surround this building falls onto the roof while I am writing this, it is likely I would be injured or even killed.

No matter how carefully we tend to our physical well-being, sooner or later all bodies end. This is a fact that we must reckon with first. Nor can the bodies of our beloved family or friends be saved. At any time, any experience can end the body, and imprint or scar the soul.

The only indisputable guarantee is that the spirit, the original identity, will always be perfectly safe. No matter what happens to the body or the soul, the spirit remains unaffected and undamaged. For we who do not yet know ourselves as spirit, who think of ourselves as body and soul, this premise may seem strange, even threatening.

The fact that we are anxious and preoccupied with our physical safety is telling. It speaks volumes about our lack of experience as spiritual beings. It points out that we are most aware of ourselves as physical bodies, rather than spirits having a physical adventure. This is a most important distinction, and herein is the solution as well as the problem.

Most of us have been misinformed about protection. Usually, in our past somewhere, we have been taught by authority figures and painful experiences, that our best protection, or defense against harm, is an overt offense. So we assume a defensive stance, attacking whatever seems threatening, even before we are attacked. This we deem necessary in order to be safe from an expected onslaught. Or we have been persuaded to rely on "outside protection," someone or something purported to be a more capable, or "stronger" champion than we. These faulty teachings do nothing but confirm our deepest fear that we are always vulnerable and unsafe because we are somehow inherently compromised or flawed. Obviously this kind of teaching has grounded us in the fearful tactics that fill the daily news.

If there could be one governing rule for masterful spiritual behavior, it would be "Never meet force with force." Force is not the almighty power of the universe. Flow is. The ultimate spiritual "powers" are manifest in us when we are in Flow, not when we have reduced ourselves to forceful, fearful attempts to control and dominate. The most powerful warrior is one who never has to draw the sword. If we would be free of the fear that makes us easy prey to what is opportunistic and harmful, then we must know we are more than just human. We must learn to be response-able rather than merely react-able. Then threat is experienced differently. When we learn that the "real" part of us cannot be threatened, and accept that the "unreal" part can only exist temporarily, we are no longer at the mercy of perceived menace. Thus invulnerability is not dependent upon conditions; body, mind, soul, and spirit live in the peace that surpasses circumstances and understanding.

Strengthening the Spiritual Immune System

Just as strengthening the physical immune system is but a temporary expedient, in that when it is time for the body to end such care is no longer required, so also is strengthening the spiritual immune system (SIS) an interim strategy. However, the SIS does not wait for death to end its viability. As soon as one begins to realize the power of the immutable original identity, the need for constant vigilance against impending doom is no longer the primary focus of the mind. Then the mind creates a much different life. Where fear in its dreadful forms once filled life's stage, now the play is delightful, even laughable.

One only need fortify the spiritual immune system while one is in training to remember the invulnerability of the original identity. This can be likened to planting zucchini in a summer garden. In the beginning the plant takes a bit of tending, but once it sprouts, there is zucchini all over the place. So it is with "re-cog-nizing," calling to mind, the capacities of the spirit. The God-Almighty Spirit that is our original nature is indomitable, impregnable, and unassailable. Now that is power!

Here is how we reawaken the sleeping giant that we truly are:

Pay Attention

Paying attention is a great and ancient spiritual mastery. Few of us have achieved any significant degree of proficiency in it. The keystone of protection is the ability to pay attention.

Most of us live in a kind of trance. We are usually running on automatic. In our overcrowded, overstressed, overstimulated lives, we are scarcely able to be aware of what we are doing today, much less recall what we did yesterday. Therein lies the problem. If we are not attentive, we are not conscious but hypnotized.

Because our attention span is so limited, we live in a kind of stupor, too often bewildered about how we got where we are, and what happened along the way. We cannot make responsible choices when entranced, because we forget we are constantly choosing, with or without awareness. If asked about our spiritual progress, we are likely to give ourselves more credit than is due because we bewitch ourselves with delusions, whether they be of grandeur or diminishment.

The simple task of observing, *and acknowledging*, which thoughts, words, emotions, and actions one is choosing, is not only life-enhancing, it creates a life of integrity. By noticing what kind of decisions and choices we make, we discover a lot about our modus operandi. We learn we have a tendency towards fearful fantasy. If the mind were not so powerfully creative this would not matter, but our minds are immensely productive. The mind is a non-stop manufacturing device. We supply the raw material, and it produces.

So the question is: What do I want to produce? When I am oblivious, it is easy for the mind to become limp, no spiritual muscles here. The absence of attention allows the mind to grow the habit of focusing on what is dark, fearful, hateful, angry, guilty, and so on. This is an open-door invitation to destruction.

Therefore, with everything I think, say, do and feel, I am *always* making a "contribution" to my life, and to humankind. I am either contributing to the light of the world, or adding to its darkness. What a (potentially) wonderful or disastrous responsibility!

Homework: Commit to paying attention one day per month. Notice how quickly you lapse into a hypnotic fog. When this happens, do not judge, condemn, or beat yourself up. Merely notice. Then make a new choice to pay attention. Choose again and again to pay attention. There is no limit on how many new choices you can make. Keep bringing yourself back to attention. If you catch yourself slipping, you are doing well, because you are paying attention.

At the end of the day take the tally of your attention quotient. Are there activities, people, conditions (driving, household chores, boring conversations, mundane tasks, eating, etc.) that contribute to your loss of attention? Are you more or less aware at certain times of the day or night? Do you resist paying attention, or refuse outright to do so?

This is helpful information to have. As you continue to flex the muscles of your spiritual immune system, your awareness will expand as you reclaim dominion in life.

The Triune Law of Right Livelihood
Thoughts, Words, and Deeds

What we think, say, and do are the raw materials of creativity. We become, or we manifest the in-kind product of our ideas, declarations, and actions. It is naive to believe we can ignore or bypass any of the three parts of these "fate makers." No amount of internal deal making will produce a different result. Despite our equivocations, "purity of thought, word, and deed" is not just for the boy scouts. If we want to enjoy peace of mind, well-being, and abundance, the laws of right livelihood must be practiced.

Thoughts

Everything originates in thought. We are a product of thought. All thoughts, our own, other people's, and the collective world thought, affect us. Thoughtforms, the byproduct of our mental clarity or mental sludge, exalt or congest our own lives and everyone else's.

Thoughts *are* things. They take form and impact our lives and the world at large. Until we fully comprehend that the power of our mind is sufficient to "create" the world we live in, we can delude ourselves into believing that so long as we are not aware what we are thinking, we will be spared the consequences of those thoughts. All thoughts have consequences that are causal in life. Ignorance of what we are creating with our thoughts is not a protection from the repercussions of those thoughts.

Christ said to pray unceasingly. Could it be that focused attention is "praying"? Especially when we "concentrate" a thought by feeling a strong emotion, we are actually praying. I wonder if Christ meant we cannot but "pray" unceasingly, since we are seldom without thought. If thought is the instrument of creation, then regardless what we claim to be thinking (or praying), we will receive as we have "asked," or thought. Therefore, questions for everyday, moment-to-moment consideration, might be "What am I 'asking' for, or 'praying' for, right now?"

"What am I 'growing' with this thought?"

"In this moment, what is the quality of my thoughts?"

"What do my thoughts demand?"

"Is this thought beneficial or is it damaging?"

All thoughts "demand" a response. The quality of the thought determines if it will either contribute to one's own well-being, and subsequently the world's well-being; or will postpone or destroy well-being. Such is the power of the God-created mind. Consequently, we must be aware what it is we are asking to receive. When we focus our thinking on what we would avoid, what we do not want, what we fear, or what is destructive, dreadful, or painful, we are *actively* praying for the unwanted to occur. Thus, our "prayerful" thought empowers those things which are contrary to well-being, or which oppose integrity of being.

It is simple to ascertain the quality of one's thinking since there are only two kinds of thought. Spiritually, energetically, psychologically, and physically, thoughts are either:

(1) positive, loving, constructive, and peaceful; or

(2) the negative, hateful, destructive, and combative.

So if one's thoughts are anxious, guilty, shameful, angry, hurtful, resistant, and so on, they do not make a contribution to well-being, no matter how we would justify them.

On the other hand, if one's thoughts are gentle, compassionate, forgiving, non-judgmental and nonviolent, they increase the flow of receiving and giving well-being. There are no exceptions to this fact. Equivocating or rationalizing will have no effect whatsoever.

So if one's "intention" is to make a positive contribution in life, but ones thoughts are not of the above mentioned category-(1) type, the intention will be overruled by the fact of in-kind consequence. In other words, believe it or not, accept it or not, life constantly shows us what we are actually thinking. Our job is to learn the truth about what is in our minds.

Homework: One day per month commit to observing your thinking. What you are looking for is fear. Of course, before we can clean up our thinking, we must first be aware how much of our thought is fear based. This is because fear in any form will obstruct and interfere with our ability to give and receive positive contributions.

An easy definition for fear is anything that is not positive, loving, constructive, or peaceful. Thus, no matter what "hat" fear is wearing, anything unlike the above definition is fear. That includes worry, anxiety, cruelty, anger, guilt, blame, shame, resentment, jealousy, and so on, are all fear wearing a different hat. If you have the desire to justify or defend the thinking, consider it fear. If you long to be right about what you are thinking, treat this as fear. "Stinking thinking" exacts a severe toll on well-being.

When you discover yourself engaged in "stinking thinking," do not chastise yourself. Simply notice. If you are like the rest of us you may discover that a large percentage of time is spent fantasizing on what is wrong in your life, or the world's horrific conditions, or what might befall you or those you love, etc. Each time you catch yourself, simply make a new choice to focus on what is lovely, or kind, compassionate, or gentle, or what is beneficial to all, but do not define how that would look. Let Love do that. If you lapse back into fear, choose again, and again, and again. It takes a while to break the habit of being held captive by fear.

At the end of the day, take account of how much time is spent "praying" fearfully. Success is catching yourself in fear, and consciously focusing on something else. So if you make ten thousand new choices in a day you are doing great!

Declarations

Words are energy. They are a powerful vibrational and tonal means of creation. Throughout antiquity "the word" was considered a sacred power to be used prudently. In ancient Greece, the pre-Socratic Stoics considered Logos to be the rational principle of the cosmos, identified with God and constituting the power of reason in the human soul. In St. John's gospel, Logos is said to be the creative word of God.[1]

We humans are favored with the conscious creative use of the spoken and written word. As part of our spiritual birthright, "the logos" is too often ignored and taken for granted. Speaking is a privilege of the conscious mind. In our daily lives we do not often consider the gift and the consequence of the spoken word. Regularly we neglect the discipline of intentional, careful use of our words. For the most part we pay little heed to what we say, how we say it, or when. Such a lackadaisical attitude regarding the *power of our declarations* has sometimes gotten us in trouble.

In days gone by, people realized that all words had issue. Agreements were contracted by a person's word. What one said had substance, and people were categorized by whether their "word" was good or bad (which meant meaningless). Now, however, we don't seem to take our words as seriously as we once did. Every day we say things without consideration of consequence. We do not mean what we say, or what we mean, we will not say. In emotional outbursts we blurt out cruel and vile words, words which compromise ourselves, and any others in their path.

This is a mistake. Words are still as potent and meaningful as ever they were; and like all volitional proclamations, enduring the consequences of our words remains a great prerogative. We can have the fruits of our pronouncements, or suffer the consequences of them.

Politicians battle with words, poets make love with words, story-tellers enchant with words. Words of wisdom uplift us. With words we bless or condemn one another. By our word(s), we reveal the state of our relationship with our divine nature, and with the Source of that nature.

Yet the use of profanity has become so pervasive that it is no longer considered an insult to polite society. Profanity has become trendy and it is fashionable to lace our conversations with words which foul the mouth and taint the mind. We no longer flinch at the vulgarity we so regularly hear. However, not so long ago scurrilous speaking and irreverent attitudes for what is sacred was not a universally accepted part of speech. No culture can afford to disregard the language of its people. We who casually adopt an obscene way of speaking are greasing the slide to our own spiritual demise. By our words, we declare it so.

For this reason, we must not allow our wounds, fears, or weaknesses to "speak" for us. Unfortunately, this is often precisely what we do. Rather than simply telling the truth "I do not feel like going out this evening," we beg off a commitment by claiming "I don't feel so well. I think I am coming down with something."

This is not just using "our word" as an excuse, it is a proclamation for making oneself sick. We make vows of pain, limitation, and death; such as, "This is to-die-for." "I will never trust (men, women, you) again." "I hate you so much I wish you were dead." We issue damaging proclamations: "Marriages don't work." "Love never lasts." "Relationships always fail." "I never succeed at anything."

Remember, the creative universe takes everything we say or think as a standing order to bring forth. It does not "do" jokes, slang, or colloquialism. Because we do not realize the power of "the word" we continue to issue "orders" we do not want filled; and so we limit or harm ourselves, and one another, by wrong use of this power. When we "call forth" wrongly, whether we are aware of what we are saying or not, we deny ourselves the power of "speaking into" what we do want. Thus do we continuously limit and divert the power of our word.

Homework: Remembering you are not on a mission to belittle yourself, commit one day per month to observing the nature of the day's declarations. Look for lies and avoidance of truth. Watch out for pronouncements that describe you as flawed, unworthy, less than what you are (or could be). Take note of "foul mouthed" speaking. Be aware how often "stinking thinking" is accompanied by "stinking speaking."

Your words are a personal advertisement for how you think of yourself. Ask yourself, "what do I want on my billboard?" Be on alert for ill-favored ways of speaking. When you catch yourself, choose to speak in a way that is befitting a God-created being. You may be amazed how powerful this can make you feel.

Actions

How many times have we heard the ancient adage: "Your actions speak louder than your words." To this we may add: "Your actions speak as loudly as your thoughts." We act out what we truly believe. So to discover what actually lingers in the mind we simply watch what we do. There are not enough good intentions or sweet words to cover up what we do. We may talk a different story, we may swear our actions are not what we *truly* intended, but nonetheless we always do what we believe, what is truly in our mindset. Our behavior will *tell* the truth about *who* we think ourselves to be, and the aftereffects are what our actions demand.

Though actions are not the primary shaper of life, they are the inseparable companion to what is. Thoughts are the noun in the "sentence" of life, and actions are the verb. Thoughts come first, actions follow, but both are creative and elicit a response. We cannot avoid what our actions produce. For example, when we think hatefully, speak hatefully, and act hatefully, we invite hate into our lives.

When we discover that some of our actions are less than whole-some, there is work to be done. Most of us, some of the time, fail to notice the discrepancy between the idealized version of oneself, and the way we live or show up in life. Like children, we have not learned when to say "yes" to ourselves, and when to say "no." Our behavioral boundaries have become compromised by loosely defined, and often ignored, bad habits. Habits of behavior are re-actions (repeated actions) that are reproduced *without responsible choice.* Aristotle said: "We are what we repeatedly do. Excellence, then, is not an act, but a choice." Since we are habitual beings, let us make habits that feed the soul rather than starve it.

It is not enough to wish for different results. We must *act* differ-ently. Remember the word "decent"? Not so long ago it was in pub-lic usage describing ordinary folk living a respectable, good life. Now the edges of acceptable conduct are more loosely defined. What was "simply not done" is no longer prescribed by the limits of common decency. The point beyond which we will not go, no longer a fixed and reliable measure, flaps uselessly in the wind of desire. "Beyond here there be dragons," the inscription on maps of old that warn of danger, could well be resurrected to remind us we are in deep water.

Oh, we can and do pretend we do not know the difference between right and wrong, but this kind of moral make believe exacts a cost from our well-being. Cause and effect simply will not be sepa-rated, no matter how hard we try to find exceptions in our case. Do right, live right. That is right livelihood.

Insanity could be defined as continuing to do the same thing while expecting a different result. Children hurt themselves this way until they finally connect the dots: "This act produces a result I do not like." Finally it registers: "Perhaps I should no longer do this." Then the hurt stops!

"To look is one thing. To see what you look at is another. To understand what you see is a third. To learn from what you under-stand is still something else. But to act on what you learn is all that really matters." Anonymous

Homework: One day per month make your words match your actions and thoughts. Yes, you read that right. When we actually state out loud what we are doing, we get an in-our-face signpost that we cannot ignore. Awareness then is unavoidable. By exposing and stating the truth about what you are doing, you will come face to face with the distorted part of yourself. It will not be able to hide behind "blind eyes" and denial. In other words, when you "speak" what you do, you are ordering yourself to take note of the "real" beliefs that linger behind the fictional beliefs.

Note particularly the "indecent" behaviors. Remember, however, you are not to beat yourself up. This is not about punishment and guilt. It is about discovery, honesty, and exercising the power of choice. Once such behavior is uncovered, consciously choose to forgive yourself and pause a moment to experience peace that is waiting to come to you. Peace will lead you "home" to the real you.

Impediments to Well-Being

Though one may be well schooled in religious dogma and ritual, most of us remain spiritually illiterate. Spiritual education has less to do with a particular set of dogmatic rules, and more to do with knowing and applying practical tools for sustaining "the good life" while facing the challenges of physicality.

We humans spiritually founder as seemingly limitless threats to well-being proliferate in the world, in ourselves and our families, and on the job. Too many of us are caught in a terrible and constant state of dread. Instead of living in present moment possibility, we worry ourselves "to death" with "what-if" thinking. Stressing in advance over what might be only adds to the world-wide body of fear.

When we "paint" with fear on the canvas of life the work we produce is not artful but awful. As we lock into imaginings of "what if," we ignore "what is," and even during the peaceful times we wait for the next alarming event to befall us. So often what we imagine is worse than what occurs. By remaining stuck in what-if apprehension, "what is next" is also shaped by fear. Remembering that we "grow" what we focus on, let us not propagate a garden of horrors.

It is simple to recognize when and if one is thinking fearfully.

The three categories of creative thought are:

1. *Fearful* that looks to the future with frightful trepidation. By arguing for "what-if" calamities, fear creates many alarming possibilities.

2. *Peaceful* that accepts "what is" in the present moment, and knows to trust that all will be well in spite of appearances.

3. *Neutral* that has neither preference nor judgment, and rests calmly while asking "what next?"

Fear

We speak now of the debilitating fears, not about the instinctual fear that rises when the body's survival is threatened. Though we may not realize it, a disproportionate amount of our time is involved in some kind of fear thought. It is shocking to discover we live as fearful primates. Fear is the single most effective tool of the dark. Without our fear the darkness would have very little influence on us.

As I see it, fear can be summarized within three main categories:

1. I will not get what I want.

2. I will lose what I have.

3. There is not enough to go around.

Honest examination of one's mindset will likely lead, directly or indirectly, to a hidden coffer of fears. Fear is a universal condition. Most times it is the great barrier to human growth. As we grow older we learn more and more fears so that by the time we reach maturity most of us are loaded with them. Some would say this is gained wisdom, but fear is seldom wise and more often ruinous to sane, calm response.

Teeming with uncertainty and change, life is one giant unknown. Unknowns generate fears. Like signing a peace accord, when we cease to make war with what we do not know, fears diminish. Eventually as we are consistent in turning fear over to peace, fears disappear. If we do not ferret out the fear, expose it and release it, the buried fear will putrefy and spread like an infection of the mind.

The trick is not to deny the presence of fear, nor to attempt to banish it by force. Admitting to fears, and acknowledging them openly, immediately diffuses some of their harmful aspects. "Confessing" this way is sufficient to unplug the emotional charge of fears that undermine calm, clear thinking. Confessing can be an intensely empowering act of self reclamation. "Unfriendlies," whether they be self saboteurs or dark force interlopers, use our secret fears and guilts as effective tools for twisting self worth into self loathing. Fear of exposure must be active in us in order for these secrets and fears to be used as a weapon against us. Therefore, self disclosure of fears and mistakes puts us squarely in the light of remembered strength and invulnerability.

Ask yourself: Am I thinking, or am I fearing? Fear is anything unlike peace, love, or well being. Therefore all worry, concern, anxiety, doubt, uneasiness, revenge, anger, guilt, blame, condemnation, resistance, and so on, is fear. No matter how slight the disturbance, it is nonetheless fear. Just as a female cannot be a little bit pregnant, so also we cannot be a little bit fearful. With our thoughts we are either "growing" fear and thereby adding to the darkness, or we are "growing" peace and thereby contributing to the light. It is that simple. That unequivocal. There is no middle ground of fear. We are either fearful, or we are peaceful.

When I am fearful, I can be harmful. When I am loving, I can be helpful. Love joins; this is healing. Fear separates; this is traumatic. What could be clearer?

After twenty-five years of dedicated practice choosing peace instead of fear, I am still amazed how quickly my mind can slip into fear fantasies. A fear fantasy is an utterly fanciful thought that materializes from the thin air of imaginary dread. I have caught myself creating a horrid outcome from nothing more than the clay of fearful fiction. "What might be" is seldom as bad as the speculations of my fearful mind. It is astounding how devoted to terror the mind can be. If left unchecked, it will always distort unlimited possibility to craft what is appalling rather than what is appealing.

I share this because we are too often impatient with ourselves when practicing mind change. The human mind has been shaped by untold eons of change, fear, and distortion. Do not expect instant gratification. The fearful mind is a tenacious adversary to well being. The key is to keep going. When you stay on the lookout for fear, and replace it with its nemesis, compassion, delight, kindness, tranquility, you are bound to succeed. Life will improve, and you will have yourself to thank for it, and that leads to gentleness and self respect. You are teaching yourself that you are worth the effort!

Homework: Ask yourself all through the day, am I fearing or am I thinking? You may be surprised to discover how often what you assume is "thinking" is actually "fearing." No matter how many times you catch yourself in fear, be thrilled over the discovery because now you can give the fear to peace.

Before retiring, take accounts: How much of my time is spent being fearful? How am I growing my fear? When am I most fearful? What triggers fear in me?

As you go to sleep remember: Peace is love gently lifting you out of fear into safekeeping.

Ignorance

As a people we don't want to hear about ignorance, because we don't like the word. First of all we assume ignorance means that we are stupid. However ignorance comes from the word ignore which means "the condition of being uneducated, unaware, or uninformed."

By our lack of attention, and because of our fear of being flawed or unworthy, we are "persuaded" to ignore a limitless amount of available information. We discount, reject, and shrug off all kinds of useful information. If we ignore, the position we are assuming is that of our rear end being exposed as our head is in the sand. When we convince ourselves, "if I refuse to believe this is happening, it cannot be happening," we add to the load of spiritual fiction that compromises our life.

What is worse, we are often involved in some form of organized, dogmatic belief system that encourages ignorance. Some of these beliefs demand that ignorance be perpetuated, so we make promises to stay ignorant, or even to proselytize ignorance.

Ignorance is second only to fear as a threat to our balance and safety. To be ignorant is to take for granted any aspect of life by relying solely on another person's say-so, believing their experience, values, beliefs, or authority to be supremely valuable, while disregarding one's own valuable experience.

Life can be simplified when we reduce it to two fundamental activities: doing and leaving undone, or in spiritual terms, learning and unlearning. When doing or leaving undone is prompted by one's own inner knowing, wisdom is gained. However, incessant doing without the promptings of spiritual guidance can leave us hopelessly striving, without any gain in personal experience. Life can be consumed by ever-more doing, until at last one realizes she can never do enough to be good enough, or sure enough, or safe enough, or accomplished enough.

Doing or learning by imitation leaves us stranded somewhere outside our own lives without any experience to guide us. Doing or learning, prompted by one's own inner urging, and embellished by experience and revelation, provides certainty from a deep, inner reality. It does not substitute the outer reality for the inner, and considers the inner knowing at least as valuable as what is perceived outwardly. This is how self respect grows, flowers, and spreads its seeds of wisdom.

Homework: Regularly pause long enough in the frenzy of doing to "look around" for the guidance and information that is always available. Be sure to look in the unexpected "places," like your heart, your still mind when it is not straining to know, spontaneous gifts of wisdom from friends and strangers, billboards, movies, books, license plates. Everything is "speaking" if you would but notice.

Pause by quiet pause, choose knowing in place of ignorance. You are never without guidance and help, and you must be still long enough to realize it is coming to you.

Denial

Many of us are products of the New Age Movement. In the 1960s we learned that we could handle everything with affirmations. We affirmed that: "Every day in every way we are getting better and better." We assumed that endlessly saying this would really have impact.

We did not know enough to do the necessary spiritual homework of preparing the mind to integrate the deeper meaning of affirmation that it may be brought forth into experience that is impactful.

Further, we learned "If I do not believe 'it' is real, 'it' is not real." This kind of spiritual shortsightedness has no protection in it. Many of us are still functioning within that framework. We would like to think we have left it behind, yet we still live as if wishing will make "it" so. This is spiritual denial and it is "slippery" in the ways it tantalizes us into believing about ourselves what is so only in potential.

When denial is nothing more than disowning what is frightening or threatening in the mind, it is no different from other forms of make-believe. Like the lion in *The Wizard of Oz*, no matter how many times he said "I do have a heart. I do! I do! I do!" his heart was not real until he tested his resolve and courageously took a stand. Then did he truly know he had a heart, and it was stalwart.

However, there is a valuable spiritual use for denial that is too often forgotten or ignored. That is to knowingly deny that anything or anyone outside oneself can truly do us harm. This form of spiritual denial rests in the unshakable knowledge that "what" we are, that is spirit, cannot be altered or affected, ever, by anyone or anything. This kind of knowing underpins the experience of spiritual invulnerability and serves us well in the dark night of the soul.

Homework: Regularly keep a sharp eye out for falsehoods that convince us of "wished for" spiritual accomplishments. Lying to oneself leaves one caught between opposing "truths." Being two-faced is a spiritual vice that teaches us not to trust ourselves. If we need to speak of our accomplishments, make them public, and be recognized for them, we probably have not achieved any noteworthy degree of mastery. Spiritual arrogance masks a doubtful heart and uncertain mind.

Indispensable Tools

Cleaning the Mindset

Interesting word, "mind-set." It describes the window through which we view life, and the world around us. The mindset is comprised of beliefs, attitudes, thoughts, judgments, assumptions, ideals, prejudices, values, and preferences. These are formed, established, accepted, and held as "truth" as dictated by life's authoritative institutions, such as family, religion, government, culture, academia, medicine, economy, and so on.

"Belief" is a currently popular label for anything that cannot be fully understood or identified. There are three kinds of belief:

1. Those we know we have.
2. Those we don't know we have.
3. Those we long for.

Belief determines perception. Through the spectacles of belief does one perceive. If beliefs are thick or compressed, they magnify. If they are soiled, they obscure or deceive. Yet if they are regularly polished by the fingers of an examining mind, they allow for new experiences based on updated information; and new experiences can be teaching tools.

The more beliefs we have the harder it is to live the way we want. Too many beliefs, and we are conflicted, confused and confounded. Often spiritual growth is sabotaged by transparent, invisible, or lost beliefs that were implanted by authority figures before one was mature enough to realize the nature and consequence of the belief.

For the most part, we are not familiar with the beliefs that are stored in the closet of the mind. Rarely do we pick through that closet of beliefs to weed out what no longer fits, to discard hand-me-downs that no longer suit, and give away what does not serve. No one taught us we are capable of being the source of our own beliefs and thoughts, and it is purposeful to align one's beliefs and actions with one's inner guidance and goals.

However, too often the mindset mandates habitual reactions to unexamined beliefs, assumptions, judgments, values, ideals, etc. Eventually these "harden" into mental, emotional, physical, and spiritual residue. These residues influence and determine the quality of our lives by concretizing misconceptions, misinterpretations, misperceptions, and misbeliefs.

Who has not had to confront a mind that is set, rock hard in its determination not to warm to a new idea, no matter how much sense it makes. I call this "Popsicle mind." "Popsicle minds" have been hard for so long that the door to the mind is frozen shut. When this condition is extreme, it can tolerate only "artificially sweetened" delusions that support its close mindedness.

Though it may appear that special measures are required to "thaw" a frozen mind, this is not so. All it takes is a little willingness to make the mind supple with one choice at a time.

What would life be like if our mindset was representative of what we actually choose to believe? Well, actually it is! Life accurately mirrors what we truly believe. We are that powerful, that skilled in actualizing our beliefs, whether we know it or not, and whether we believe it or not. That being the case, it behooves us to become familiar with what we warehouse within the belief "system."

What would we be like if our mindset became a mind-in-flow? If we put aside rigidity and updated and regularly renewed the mind? What if we chose to be guided by perennial inner wisdom of the soul? What if?

Homework: Twice per year, New Year's Day and your birthday, spend half a day "cleaning out" the closet of the mind. Get rid of what is outdated, outworn, useless, inappropriate, and does not fit anymore.

Companions on the Road to Wholeness

Accountability and Responsibility

Somewhere along the way to remembering what we are, we lost or put aside our response-ability and instead we opted for react-ability. That is, for whatever reason, we do not respond to what is currently happening, but instead we continue to react to what happened in the past as though it was happening now. It is as if we carry the past forward and plunk it down in the present. In this way we continuously revisit or reexperience the hurts, mistakes, and perils of the past. Thus do we condemn ourselves to relive what is destructive, rather than creating anew in the present. Re-action is automatic, response is choosing in the present moment, with awareness.

Eventually this is habit forming, and we are no longer response-able but are only react-able. In this way the exquisite privilege of choice is lost to us, since we can only choose when we are "in response."

Put another way then, responsibility is being able to respond *so as to be the source or cause of what is preferable and helpful in life, now, in this moment.* Since we are always "sourcing" or "causing" something, the question becomes: sourcing or causing *what.*

Being accountable means that I am answerable for my choices. In other words, I accept the consequences of my choices. Further I realize it is likely I shall be "called to account" for my choices. Such is the groundwork of wise stewardship.

This great spiritual privilege we would cast away imagining we could then be free of liability. Such short-sightedness misses the point. As long as one is accountable, the choice, the event, and the consequence are inseparable. Therefore, one is never "under the thumb" of an outside authority. One is self determined, able to correct, heal and recreate anew rather than remain controlled and enslaved by what one sees as a greater authority than herself. The misunderstanding and misuse of authority and accountability keeps us imprisoned in powerlessness and ineffectuality. We have a choice. If the "choice" muscle has grown flaccid with misuse or lack of use, then exercise it.

We are all graced with opportunities to demonstrate spiritual, mental, emotional, and physical competence. How, or if, we maximize these opportunities is up to us. Secreted in each and every situation, including the most mundane and ordinary, is the potential to be high-minded. If we choose to ignore the opportunity, then we have missed the point of experience.

We humans want all the liberties and freedoms of the masterful, but we don't want the accountability. It behooves us to first look only to ourselves for all problems and all solutions. Radical responsibility brings radical power. If there's a problem here, I caused it. This is how we realize the solutions are here, with us, where the problems are.

Finally liberated from the Nazi death camps, Dr. Viktor Frankl came to New York and eventually traveled to California. After visiting America, Dr. Frankl said he never could understand how we could have a Statue of Liberty on the east coast without a "Statue of Responsibility" on the west coast.

Homework: Adopt the attitude: If there is a problem in my life, the common denominator is I am always at the scene of the "accident." If I see a problem, I am in the problem, I am an undeniable part of it. Viewing problems from this perspective can change one's life. Now what am I going to do about it? Make a different choice!

Authority

"Response-ableness" is a blessing, not a curse, and not a duty. It is by being response-able that we claim our authority, that is to author our own lives. To be deprived of the privilege of response-ableness is to always be controlled by some outside authority; someone or something which is bigger, stronger, more powerful, holier, etc., than we. To turn away from response-ableness is to disclaim our original nature, and thereby "slide sideways" into thinking ourselves as less than we were created to be.

We of this generation, certainly in the West, are determined to assign authorship of life to something outside of ourselves. We insist on it in most aspects of life. We deify the institutions in our society until our experience is really dominated by authority figures (parents, teachers, doctors, ministers/priests, police, lawyers, politicians, the powers that be), situations, circumstances, crises, and so on. Thereby we continue to give over our power to someone or something else until we are finally "out of control." Thus we give away dominion by relinquishing self control. It would seem we really don't mind paying the price of being without sovereignty, so long we do not have to be the responsible authority in our own life. The buck no longer stops here; it gets passed along to whichever "tyrant" will snatch it up.

This kind of subjective relinquishment of power is not limited to physical life. We do it in our spiritual life as well when we look for something outside of ourselves to make "it" better. Even when we talk about the "spirit within" what we almost always mean is the "spirit without." Our inner looking is actually looking out for the answer, a looking out for the *deus ex machina*, a "helper from heaven." Rarely do we trust that help can come from within one's own "be-ing-ness," or the holiness within which is our true nature.

No being of light will do for us what is our privilege to do for ourselves. Why? Because to do so is to discredit we who believe we are less than able, and therefore add to the measure of imagined helplessness. This is not to say there is not help from the divine. It is to clarify that help comes in teaching mode rather than doing-for mode. Beings of light teach us to be self sufficient that we may remember we are children of light. Like all children we whine for someone "greater" to do "it" for us. Yet a good "parent" always helps us to learn how to do "it" for ourselves. This is not cruelty. It is love.

Homework: Allow the body to tell you what the mind refuses to say. Pay attention to the bodily signals (goosebumps, thrills, prickles, tingles, sighs, racing heart, change in breathing, and so on) that indicate something worth noting is happening. The body is a great communicator and it often recognizes what the mind discounts. You do not make this earthly journey alone. Mighty companions are always with you. You may be oblivious to all kinds of guidance and assistance. Pay attention—and ask for help.

Discipline

Note: Before we go further I will tell you of a spiritual choice I long ago made. That is, for me, the divine is exemplified by the Holy Spirit. I chose this feminine aspect of the divine (1) because of the interface the Holy Spirit has with Earth and we humans; and (2) because of the qualities of the Holy Spirit. In my experience the Holy Spirit is the guide, caretaker, nurturer, advocate, and teacher. Also the Holy Spirit helps me make corrections, and gives succor, sanctuary, solace, and comfort. The Holy Spirit is with me as I journey through life. I abide and rest in the Holy Spirit.

I share this not to influence your choice but to clarify mine.

Most of us do not much like discipline. It asks too much of us. After all, we are "free spirits" with "free will" who do not want anyone telling us what to do or how to do it. Yet without discipline, that is the "training expected to produce a specific character or pattern of behavior, especially training that produces moral or mental improvement"[2] spiritual awareness will not develop. Regardless which spiritual philosophy we choose, by discipline is meant the daily, regular, ongoing commitment to "still" the "monkey mind" and make an experiential connection to that which is holy, or beyond the distractions of finite physical life.

The core word in discipline is "disciple." To be a disciple means to be "an active adherent." We are being asked to actively initiate and maintain a relationship with the divine. This is just like cultivating a relationship with a would-be friend. The first step in sustaining a good friendship is keeping in touch. It is exactly the same with God.

It does not matter what we call that which is sacred—Holy Spirit, Universal Mind, higher self, inner knower, God, angels, divine mother, or the heart. What matters is that we connect with It, and are intimate with It. The form this connection takes is not as important as sustaining the relationship. Whether we think of this as meditation, contemplation, prayer, or communication, regardless what we call It, we must make contact. Then we must "grow" this relationship. What is needed is more than a fleeting or occasional nod towards the divine. It is not sufficient to only cry for help while ignoring God all the other times. This bond has to be as vital and juicy, as personal and unlimited as the river that flows between beloveds.

Realize that lack of concentration is not the only problem we have with discipline. Rather it is our misbelief that none of us, especially oneself, is (really) worth the consistent vigilance that spiritual discipline demands. This is one of our worst self deceptions: the deeply disguised and disheartening belief that we are, at our core, flawed and therefore not worth the effort it takes to rebuild our spiritual awareness. *In every case of spiritual self deception, the problem is always we have thought wrongly about what we are.*

Homework: Begin with only five minutes in the morning, and five minutes in the evening. Set aside this time to simply "tune into" the stillness that is already present inside oneself. This is more a "not doing" than a "doing." Stillness is there. Peace and calm are there. Persevere. Make contact.

Witnessing

Along with forgiveness, "right witnessing" is perhaps our most important function as citizens of a spiritually sick world. We can only be healers one for another when we *insist* on seeing everyone as spiritually worthy, in spite of all appearances to the contrary. This "spiritual service" is especially crucial when one is temporarily unable to do this for oneself. There are times when people lose touch with their original nature. To remember for another when she is in the pits of darkness, be it a spiritual, mental, emotional, or physical crisis, is how we function as agents of repair for each other, and for the entire world. "Holding" someone as light while they cannot do this for themselves can be an immense relief. Plus it is profoundly healing just to know someone would do this.

"Holding as light" is as simple as imagining or visualizing the person awash with light. Keep in mind the image of that person as light. Look right past any appearances to the contrary. Mentally insist on maintaining the picture of them as filled to overflowing with bright, clear, white light. Whenever they come to mind, see them this way. One cannot do this too often for themselves, for another, and for the world. Humans are desperately in need of this kind of radiant, loving care of one another.

What seems to be an unlikely theory is supported by the work of Rupert Sheldrake, a British scientist. In his theory of morphogenetic fields he offers fascinating evidence that once enough people embrace an idea it achieves sufficient persuasive power to influence others at large. We have heard of this as the "Hundredth Monkey" principle.

What exciting possibilities this portends! A spiritual grass-roots movement to compassionately hold all humans as light. Whether manifesting as light or something less, not one of us is to be left behind. Such spiritual generosity could actually lift humankind out of the dregs irreconcilable cruelty. Remember: We are always contributing to the light or the dark.

Homework: Practice holding another as light, especially when you have judged them otherwise; or when they are temporarily forgetful of their own original nature; or when they appear to be unworthy of such kindness. (Especially do this with yourself. We are harsh and often merciless with our own "little" frightened selves.)

For Correction of Errors

Forgiveness

Though misunderstood, forgiveness is perhaps the greatest healing tool on Earth, and the most efficient means for keeping us in successful relationship with life.

Unfortunately most of us have been taught wrongly about forgiveness. Consequently, too few have a true understanding of forgiveness and are therefore deprived of its far-reaching benefits.

There is a way to forgive that leaves everyone feeling like they've won. Contrary to what "churchianity" has taught about forgiveness, it is not about someone from a lofty, righteous position looking down upon a lowly, ne'er-do-well, and deigning to bestow pardon and mercy.

Forgiveness is not what some therapists are wont to do. That is, to endlessly repeat the "processing" of grievances, thereby bringing them forward from the past into the present where they can continue to taint the life one could be living now.

Neither is forgiveness the New Age habit of burying unresolved injuries and injustices under sugar-coated affirmations. Pretending to let the hurt go only insures it will fester and resurface more virulently at some other inopportune time.

Forgiveness is never about disowning one's deeply felt injuries; nor does it make believe that heinous behavior did not occur. Forgiveness neither denies crime, injustice, or atrocity nor does it condone. What forgiveness does is bring relief from the pain, grief, and paralysis of injury. Real or imagined, injury *feels* the same. Therefore forgiveness does not necessarily attempt to psychoanalyze what is so for the ones who suffer. Rather it simply makes what hurts go away.

Forgiveness, more than anything else, chips away at, and finally disappears, the fear and darkness hiding in our minds and hearts that it may not continue to poison life. Wherever unforgiveness is lurking there will also likely be guilt, anger, blame, shame, and the desire for revenge. These destructive emotions lay out a welcome mat for the onslaught of a multitude of anti-life energies. Whether the unforgiveness frees another or oneself, the gift of forgiveness places a protective and comforting "Band-Aid" over the parts of the psyche that have been injured and scarred.

However, we can't "do" forgiveness by ourselves. The truth is we need help to forgive. If we are still "hot and suffering," or if we have "cooled down and hardened," we may be blinded to the larger view of what is happening, why it is occurring, and how to escape the perplexing tangle of it. We need the exquisite clarity of the Inner Teacher who sees what is good for all and knows how to implement it. When we turn to the Inner Teacher to help us to forgive, we are tutored in mind, heart, and soul healing. Thus does forgiveness heal the scars of the soul, the broken heart, and the mistakes of the mind, that we may be saved from repeating the fearsome patterns unforgiveness evokes.

Here are the basic steps of forgiveness:

1. *Recognize* you have a problem. You are caught in the cycle of anger, guilt, accusation, projection, and futility.

2. *Be willing* that forgiveness *could* occur—in spite of yourself. No matter how impossible or unlikely this may seem. (This step is immensely helpful when you are still "bleeding" from the wound.)

3. *Acknowledge* that it does not feel good to live like this. There must be a better way.

4. *Call to the Holy Spirit for help.* Say "Give me another way to see this."

5. *Gladly accept* the new "pictures" of what happened, what it was for, what effect it has had, what it means for the future. In other words, be willing to accept that there is (or might be) another way to see this. You may not know what it is, but it is possible. (If you honestly cannot yet accept any new perspective, at least include the new ones with your own perspective.)

6. *Give over* the desire for vengeance, or justice, or vindication to the Holy Spirit. Literally hand it over. Get rid of it.

7. *Take a moment to receive* the peaceful relief that surely comes.

Homework: Practice forgiveness as soon as you notice you are "out of love," any time you feel fear in any form. Forgiveness can be as immediate as your willingness to call for help. The greatest news of all is, it is not we who "do" forgiveness. It is the Holy Spirit. So if you are feeling "I cannot forgive," be aware that is the truth. Your job is to be willing that forgiveness is possible, to accept that something else besides what you experienced could have happened, and to look at what that might be as it comes to you. All the rest is in the "hands" of the Holy Spirit.

Undoing the Consequences

This technique is another effective healing agent for the correction of "insanities" (and all forms of fear are insane), and the undoing of the consequences. As soon as possible after a mistake, misthought, mishap, ask the Holy Spirit within to help you undo the consequences of your fearful thoughts. Then name the particular error of mind or fear, and describe it briefly.

"I ask the Holy Spirit within to help me undo the consequences of my insane thought about _____. Thank You." (Gratitude is a major transformative power.)

The power of our connection with the Holy Spirit is unlimited. We can reach into the past, present, or future, and get help cleaning up the "messes" our disturbed thinking or troubled behavior may have made. Should we slip into revisiting or reclaiming our fearful thoughts by recalling them, simply repeat the process. Fortunately we are allotted an unlimited number of "undoings."

Homework: As often as necessary, undo the consequences of mistakes by calling them back and collapsing the thought bubble (like in cartoons) that would become a potential damaging thought form.

I have seen this effect miraculous corrections. The stories from people who use it are remarkable.

Try it. It takes the sting out of being "only human," and fortifies the experience of being so much more.

Summary

We adorn our bodies with crystals, amulets, medals, thinking they will bring power and protection. We cling to objects believing they will ward off an attack. We attend ceremonies and perform rituals hoping they will save us from the dark, when all the time it is in our own minds.

Ninety-five percent of all our problems would already be tended to if we were to live as though we recognize what we are, and by our mindset we are either strengthening or weakening the Spiritual Immune System. There really is so little for us to do, and so very much for us to remember. Invulnerability is always about being; protection is about heeding.

If we will ask ourselves: "Does this thought/opinion/action add to the light or darkness of this world?" then we can make a difference, in our own life and in the world. *We are always contributing to the light or to the darkness.* We are either the instruments of repair we are meant to be, or we are being used as tools of destruction.

We cannot seek after mastery while neglecting its basic requirements. Though we sometimes believe ourselves inadequate to the task, this basic spiritual curriculum is not too difficult for us to master for "ye [we] are gods."

We are perfectly safe divine beings of light, manifesting love as life. We are already, always, in full possession of invincible invulnerability. What we lack is the awareness of our original identity. It is the inability or refusal to "know thySelf" that deprives us of the gifts of our spiritual heritage. We are, by our own hand, co-makers of our travails. We cannot but be what we were created to be. No matter what. No exceptions. However, we must realize what that is. And we must accept it. We are now, and will always be, the holy, and therefore safe, children of the God.

And that is protection.

Appendix C
Sealing Light Meditation

Focus deep inside to the very center of your being. Find your own spark of Light there, your own spark of God consciousness, your connection to Creator Source. Feel it, see it, sense it there, imagine it there, deep within you. Imagine the spark of Light as it spreads through your soul, into your body, glowing warmly and expanding in every direction, upward and downward. The Light expands all the way from the tips of your toes to the top of your head, across your shoulders, down your arms, from fingertips to fingertips, filling every cell of your physical body. Imagine the Light expanding outward beyond the boundaries of your body about an arm's length in every direction. On either side, over your head and beneath your feet, in front of you, and especially behind you. Our physical eyes focus forward and we tend to ignore our back. Imagine a shimmering bubble of golden white Light all around you. Remember the Light often, when you go to sleep, when you awaken, every time you smile, every time you breathe, each time your heart beats. Soon it will be with you permanently.

Appendix D

False Memory Syndrome

The false memory syndrome has emerged in recent years surrounded by adverse publicity and with devastating results. There have been cases of ostensible child abuse, recalled in therapy by an adult client who then brings legal action against the suspected abusers, usually parents. In some cases, it has been shown that the suspected events could not have possibly occurred. This is a tragic situation, and there is no obvious solution.

Skeptical critics of regression therapy, past-life therapy, spirit releasement therapy, soul fragment recovery, and therapy for any kind of UFO contact or abduction experience will point to the evidence of false memories. Such debunkers callously ignore the pain, the confusion, the obvious distress of clients who suffer the residue of past trauma, entity attachment, or UFO interaction, and label it imagination. This is a terrible disservice to people who have suffered such trauma.

At least one state has attempted to restrict therapy by criminalizing the use of any events retrieved from memory. It would effectively destroy any possibility of therapeutic intervention by psychotherapists.

It is not unusual for a client in altered state to "recall" symptoms usually associated with memories of being aborted, yet the trauma belongs to the attached entity of an unborn child who was aborted. "Memories" of sexual abuse can be uncovered, as can memories of cult abuse. It doesn't mean the abuse didn't happen; the memories belong to someone else who is no longer living. Release of the attached entities erases the trauma of the memories. Such memories can also be carried from former lifetimes. There are specific techniques to make the differential diagnosis.

Some memories can be suggested by an eager interrogator who offers multiple choice questions to the person in an altered state of consciousness. The interrogator has an agenda and wants the subject to come up with the "right" answers. The human mind is highly suggestible.

It is interesting and distressing to note that the legal system relies heavily on testimony by witnesses who call on memory, sometimes years after the event they are describing. How many people have been executed because of one witness's false memory? The possibilities are appalling.

Bibliography

Abrams, Jeremiah. (1990). *Reclaiming the Inner Child.* Los Angeles: Jeremy P. Tarcher.

Ader, Robert, David Felton, and Nicholas Cohen. (1991). *Psychoneuroimmunology,* Second Edition. San Diego: Academic Press.

Alexander, Marc. (1978). *The Man Who Exorcised the Bermuda Triangle.* New York: A. S. Barnes.

Allison, Ralph. (1980). *Minds in Many Pieces.* New York: Rawson, Wade.

American Psychiatric Association. (1994). *Diagnostic and Statistical Manual of Mental Disorders,* Fourth Edition. Washington, D.C.: Author.

Anshen, Ruth Nanda. (1972). *The Reality of the Devil: Evil in Man.* New York: Delta.

Ashley, Leonard R. N. (1996). *The Complete Book of Devils and Demons.* New York: Barricade.

Assagioli, Robert. (1965). *Psychosynthesis.* New York: Viking.

Atwater, P. M. H. (1994). *Beyond the Light.* New York: Carol Publishing Group.

Avery, Jeanne. (1996). *A Soul's Journey.* Austin, Tex.: Boru Books.

Baldwin, William. (1988). *Diagnosis and Treatment of the Spirit Posses-sion Syndrome.* Unpublished doctoral dissertation, American Commonwealth University, San Diego.

————. (1992). *Spirit Releasement Therapy: A Technique Manual,* Second Edition. Terra Alta, W. Va.: Headline Books.

Barlow, D., G. Abel, and E. Blanchard, (1977). "Gender Identity Change in a Transsexual: An Exorcism." *Archives of Sexual Behav-ior,* Vol. 6 (pp. 387–395).

Basham, Don. (1972). *Deliver Us from Evil.* Washington Depot, Conn.: Chosen Books.

Berne, Eric. (1961). *Transactional Analysis in Psychotherapy.* New York: Grove.

————. (1978). *Games People Play.* New York: Ballantine.

Bernstein, Morey. (1956). *The Search for Bridey Murphy.* New York: Doubleday.

Blatty, William P. (1971). *The Exorcist.* New York: Harper & Row.

Bletzer, June. (1986). *The Donning International Encyclopedic Psychic Dictionary.* Norfolk, Va.: The Donning Company.

Bradshaw, John. (1990). *Homecoming: Reclaiming and Championing Your Inner Child.* New York: Bantam.

Bramley, William. (1993). *Gods of Eden.* New York: Avon.

Brandon, Ruth. (1983). *The Spiritualists: The Passion for the Occult in the Nineteenth and Twentieth Centuries.* New York: Alfred A. Knopf.

Braun, B. G. (Ed.). (1986). *Treatment of Multiple Personality Disorder.* Washington, D.C.: American Psychiatric Press.

Brennan, Barbara Ann. (1987). *Hands of Light: A Guide to Healing through the Human Energy Field.* New York: Bantam.

Brittle, Gerald. (1980). *The Demonologist.* Englewood Cliffs, N. J.: Prentice Hall.

Bruyere, Rosalyn. (1989). *Wheels of Light: A Study of the Chakras.* Sierra Madre, Calif.: Bon Productions.

Budge, E. A. Wallis. (1967). *Egyptian Book of the Dead.* New York: Dover.

Bull, Titus. (1932). *Analysis of Unusual Experience in Healing Relative to Diseased Minds.* New York: James H. Hyslop Foundation.

Campbell, Joseph (Ed.). (1976). *The Portable Jung.* New York: Penguin.

Campbell, Robert J. (Ed.). (1981). *Psychiatric Dictionary,* Fifth Edition. New York: Oxford University.

Cerminara, Gina. (1950) *Many Mansions.* New York: Sloane.

Chamberlain, D. (1988). *Babies Remember Birth: Extraordinary Scientific Discoveries About the Mind and Personality of Your Newborn.* Los Angeles: Tarcher.

Chaplin, Annabel. (1977). *The Bright Light of Death.* Marina del Rey, Calif.: DeVorss.

Clare, Maryanne. (1997). *The Splintered Soul: Shamanic Journeys to Heal the Inner Darkness.* Santa Fe: Heartsfire Books.

Coleman, J. C., J. N. Butcher, and R. C. Carlson. (1980). *Abnormal Psychology and Modern Life,* Sixth Edition. Glenview, Ill.: Scott, Foresman & Company.

Cox, D. (1968). *Modern Psychology: The Teachings of Carl Gustav Jung.* New York: Harper & Row.

Crabtree, Adam. (1993). *From Mesmer to Freud.* New Haven: Yale University Press.

———. (1997). *Multiple Man.* Toronto: Somerville House.

———. (1997). *Trance Zero: Breaking the Spell of Conformity.* Toronto: Somerville House.

Crampton, Martha. (1981). "Psychosynthesis." In R. Corsini (Ed.), *Handbook of Innovative Psychotherapies.* (pp. 709–723). New York: Wiley.

Cranston, Sylvia, and Carey Williams. (1984). *Reincarnation: A New Horizon In Science, Religion, and Society.* New York: Julian.

Deutsch, David, Ph.D. (1997). *The Fabric of Reality.* Great Britain: Penguin Books Ltd.

Dilts, Robert, John Grinder, Richard Bandler, Leslie Bandler, Judith DeLozier. (1980). *Neuro-Linguistic Programming: Vol. 1, The Study of the Structure of Subjective Experience.* Cupertino, Calif.: Meta Publications.

Dossey, Larry. (1993). *Healing Words: The Power of Prayer and the Practice of Medicine.* San Francisco: HarperSanFrancisco.

Ellenberger, Henri F. (1970). *The Discovery of the Unconscious: The History and Evolution of Dynamic Psychiatry.* New York: Basic Books.

Feher, Leslie. (1981). *The Psychology of Birth: Roots of Human Personality.* New York: Continuum.

Fenimore, Angie. (1995). *Beyond the Darkness.* New York: Bantam.

Ferrucci, Piero. (1982). *What We May Be.* Los Angeles: Tarcher.

Finch, W. J. (1975). *The Pendulum and Possession,* Revised Edition. Sedona, Ariz.: Esoteric Publications.

Fiore, Edith. (1978). *You Have Been Here Before: A Psychologist Looks at Past Lives.* New York: Ballantine.

———. (1987a). *The Unquiet Dead: A Psychologist Treats Spirit Possession.* New York: Doubleday/Dolphin.

———. (1987b, September). "The Unquiet Dead." Lecture presented at the Seventh Annual Fall Conference of the Association for Past-Life Research and Therapy, Sacramento, Calif.

———. (1989). *Encounters: A Psychologist Reveals Case Studies of Abductions by Extraterrestrials.* New York: Doubleday.

Fodor, Nandor. (1949). *The Search for the Beloved: A Clinical Investigation of the Trauma of Birth and Pre-Natal Conditioning.* New York: Hermitage.

Foulks, E. (1985). In B. O'Regan (Ed.), *Investigations: Research Bulletin of the Institute of Noetic Sciences.* Vol. 1, No. 3/4 (p. 7). Sausalito, Calif.: IONS.

Fremantle, F., and C. Trungpa (1975). *The Tibetan Book of the Dead.* Boulder, Colo.: Shambhala.

Friesen, James. (1991). *Uncovering the Mystery of MPD: Its Shocking Origins . . . Its Surprising Cure.* San Bernardino, Calif.: Here's Life.

Gabriel, Michael. (1992). *Voices from the Womb.* Lower Lake, Calif.: Aslan.

Gallup, George. (1982). *Adventures in Immortality.* New York: McGraw-Hill.

Gauld, Alan. (1968). *The Founders of Psychical Research.* New York: Schocken Books.

Gershom, Rabbi Yonassan. (1992). *Beyond the Ashes: Cases of Reincarnation from the Holocaust.* Virginia Beach: A.R.E. Press.

———. (1996). *From Ashes to Healing: Mystical Encounters with the Holocaust.* Virginia Beach: A.R.E. Press.

Greene, Brian. (1999). *The Elegant Universe.* New York: Vintage Books.

Grof, Stanislov. (1975). *Realms of the Human Unconscious: Observations from LSD Research.* New York: Viking Press.

Grof, Stanislov, and Joan Halifax. (1976). "Psychedelics and the Experience of Death," in Arnold Toynbee (Ed.), *Life After Death.* (pp. 197–198). New York: McGraw-Hill.

Grof, Stanislov, and Christina Grof. (1980). *Beyond Death: The Gates of Consciousness.* New York: Thames and Hudson.

Grof, Stanislov. (1985). *Beyond the Brain: Birth, Death and Transcendence in Psychotherapy.* New York: State University of New York.

Guirdham, Arthur. (1982). *The Psychic Dimensions of Mental Health.* Great Britain: Turnstone.

Hall, Calvin, and Vernon. S. Nordby. (1973). *A Primer of Jungian Psychology.* New York: New American Library.

Hall, Calvin. (1979). *A Primer of Freudian Psychology*, 25th Anniversary Edition. New York: New American Library.

Hammond, Ida Mae and Frank Hammond. (1973). *Pigs in the Parlor: A Practical Guide to Deliverance.* Kirkwood, Mo.: Impact Books.

Harner, Michael. (1980). *The Way of the Shaman.* San Francisco: Harper & Row.

Hastings, Arthur. (1991). *With the Tongues of Men and Angels: A Study of Channeling.* Fort Worth, Tex.: Holt, Rinehart and Winston.

Head, J., and S. Cranston. (1967). *Reincarnation in World Thought.* New York: Julian.

———. (1977). *Reincarnation: The Phoenix Fire Mystery.* New York: Julian.

———. (Eds.). (1999). *Reincarnation: An East-West Anthology.* White Plains: Aeon. (original work published 1961)

Hendin, H., and A. P. Haas. (1984). *Wounds of War: The Psychological Aftermath of Combat in Vietnam.* New York: Basic Books.

Herbert, Nick. (1987). *Quantum Reality: Beyond the New Physics.* New York: Anchor.

Herzog, James. (2001). *Father Hunger: Explorations with Adults and Children.* Oakland, Calif.: Analytic Press.

Hickman, Irene. (1994). *Remote Depossession.* Kirksville, Mo.: Hickman Systems.

Howe Jr., Quincy. (1974). *Reincarnation for the Christian.* Wheaton, Ill.: The Theosophical Publishing House.

Hoyt, Olga. (1978). *Exorcism.* New York: Franklin Watts.

Hyslop, James. (1920). *Contact with the Other World*. New York: The Century Co.

Ingerman, Sandra. (1991). *Soul Retrieval*. San Francisco: HarperSanFrancisco.

———. (1993). *Welcome Home*. San Francisco: HarperSanFrancisco.

James, William. (1950). *The Principles of Psychology, Vol. 1 & 2*. New York: Dover. (First published in Canada in 1890 by General Publishing Company, Ltd.)

———. (1966). In N. Fodor, *Encyclopedia of Psychic Science*. Secaucus, N.J.: The Citadel Press.

Janov, Arthur. (1983). *Imprints: The Lifelong Effects of the Birth Experience*. New York: Coward-McCann.

Kardec, Allan. (1976). *The Spirits' Book*. (Anna Blackwell, Trans.). New York: Arno Press. (original work published 1875)

———. (1977). *The Mediums' Book*. (Anna Blackwell, Trans.). London: Psychic Press. (original work published 1876)

Kelsey, Denys, and Joan Grant. (1967). *Many Lifetimes*. New York: Doubleday.

Keyes, Dan. (1981). *The Minds of Billy Milligan*. New York: Bantam.

Klimo, Jon. (1987). *Channeling: Investigations on Receiving Information From Paranormal Sources*. Los Angeles: Tarcher.

Kluft, Richard. P. (Ed.). (1985). *Childhood Antecedents of Multiple Personality*. Washington, D.C.: American Psychiatric Press.

———. (1986). "Treating Children Who Have Multiple Personality Disorder." In B. G. Braun (Ed.). *Treatment of Multiple Personality Disorder* (pp. 79–105). Washington, D.C.: American Psychiatric Press.

Kroger, William S. (1977). *Clinical and Experimental Hypnosis*, Second Edition. Philadelphia: Lippincott.

Kübler-Ross, E. (1969). *On Death and Dying*. New York: MacMillan.

Long, M. F. (1948). *The Secret Science Behind Miracles*. Marina del Rey, Calif.: DeVorss & Co.

———. (1953). *The Secret Science at Work*. Marina del Rey, Calif.: DeVorss & Co.

———. (1955). *Growing Into Light*. Marina del Rey, Calif.: DeVorss & Co.

———. (1959). *Psychometric Analysis*. Marina Del Rey, Calif.: DeVorss & Co.

————. (1976). *Alternate Realities: The Search for the Full Human Being.* New York: Ballantine.

Leboyer, Frederick. (1976). *Birth Without Violence.* New York: Alfred A. Knopf.

Leir, Dr. Roger. (1998). *The Aliens and the Scalpel.* Columbus, N.C.: Granite Publishing.

LeShan, Lawrence. (1974). *The Medium, the Mystic, and the Physicist: Toward a General Theory of the Paranormal.* New York: Viking.

Levenkron, Steven. (1982). *Treating and Overcoming Anorexia Nervosa.* New York: Scribner's.

Lewis, C. S. (1982). *The Screwtape Letters: A Devil's Diabolical Advice for the Capturing of the Human Heart.* New York: Bantam. (original work published 1942)

Linn, Matthew, and Dennis Linn. (1981). *Deliverance Prayer.* New York: Paulist Press.

MacDonald, J. (1964). "Suicide and Homicide by Automobile." *American Journal of Psychiatry,* 121 (pp. 366–370).

MacNutt, Francis. (1974). *Healing.* Notre Dame, Ind.: Ave Maria Press.

————. (1995). *Deliverance from Evil Spirits: A Practical Manual.* Grand Rapids, Mich.: Chosen Books.

Manning, Matthew, (1973). *The Link: The Extraordinary Gifts of a Teenage Psychic.* Gerrards Cross, Buckinghamshire, England: Colin Smythe.

Martin, Asa. (1942). *Researches in Reincarnation and Beyond.* Sharon, Penn.: A. R. Martin.

Martin, Malachi. (1976). *Hostage to the Devil.* New York: Bantam.

Maurey, Eugene. (1988). *Exorcism.* West Chester, Penn.: Whitford.

McAll, Kenneth. (1982). *Healing the Family Tree.* London: Sheldon.

McGee, Robert. (1993). *Father Hunger.* Ann Arbor: Vine Book— Servant Publications.

McMoneagle, Joseph. (1993). *Mind Trek: Exploring Consciousness, Time, and Space through Remote Viewing.* Charlottesville, Va.: Hampton Roads.

Meek, George. (1980). *After We Die, What Then?* Franklin, N.C.: Metascience.

Mishlove, Jeffrey. (1975). *Roots of Consciousness: Psychic Liberation through History, Science and Experience*. New York: Random House and Bookworks.

Modi, Shakuntala, M.D. (1997). *Remarkable Healings: A Psychiatrist Discovers Unsuspected Roots of Mental and Physical Illness*. Charlottesville, Va.: Hampton Roads.

Monroe, Robert. (1971). *Journeys Out of the Body*. New York: Doubleday.

———. (1985). *Far Journeys*. Garden City, N.Y.: Doubleday/Dolphin.

———. (1994). *The Ultimate Journey*. N.Y.: Doubleday.

Montgomery, John Warwick (Ed.). (1976). *Demon Possession*. Minneapolis: Bethany Fellowship, Inc.

Montgomery, Ruth. (1979). *Strangers Among Us*. New York: Ballantine.

Moustakas, Clark. (1990). *Heuristic Research: Design, Methodology, and Applications*. Newbury Park, Calif.: Sage.

Myers, F. W. H. (1904). *Human Personality and Its Survival of Bodily Death* in two volumes. New York: Longmans, Green, & Co.

Myss, Caroline. (1996). *Anatomy of the Spirit: The Seven Stages of Power and Healing*. New York: Harmony.

Naegeli-Osjord, Hans. (1988). *Possession and Exorcism*. (S. and D. Coats, Trans.). Oregon, Wis.: New Frontiers Center. (original work published 1983)

Nauman, St. Elmo. (1974). *Exorcism through the Ages*. Secaucus, N.J.: Citadel.

Netherton, Morris. (1978). *Past Lives Therapy*. New York: William Morrow.

Newton, Michael. (1995). *Journey of Souls*. St. Paul, Minn.: Llewellyn Publications.

———. (2000). *Destiny of Souls*. St. Paul, Minn.: Llewellyn Publications.

Nicola, Rev. John. (1974). *Diabolical Possession And Exorcism*. Rockford, Ill.: Tan Books.

Oesterreich, Trauggot. (1974). *Possession and Exorcism*. (D. Ibberson, Trans.) New York: Causeway. (original work published 1921)

Peck, M. Scott. (1983). *People of the Lie*. New York: Simon & Schuster.

Penfield, Wilder, M.D. (1975). *The Mystery of the Mind*. Princeton, N.J.: Princeton University Press.

Pert, Candace. (1997). *Molecules of Emotion: Why You Feel the Way You Feel.* New York: Scribner.

Putnam, F. (1985). In B. O'Regan (Ed.), *Investigations: Research Bulletin of the Institute of Noetic Sciences.* Vol. 1, No. 3/4 (p. 11). Sausalito, Calif.: IONS.

Putnam, Frank. (1989). *Diagnosis and Treatment of Multiple Personality Disorder.* New York: Guilford.

Rama, S., R. Ballentine, and S. Ajaya. (1976). *Yoga and Psychotherapy.* Honesdale, Penn.: The Himalayan Institute of Yoga Science and Philosophy.

Ravenscroft, Trevor. (1973). *The Spear of Destiny: The Occult Power Behind the Spear Which Pierced the Side of Christ.* York Beach, Maine: Weiser.

Ravenscroft, Trevor, and Tim Wallace-Murphy. (1997). *The Mark of the Beast.* York Beach, Maine: Weiser.

Rawlings, Maurice. (1993). *To Hell and Back.* Nashville: Thomas Nelson.

Reed, Anderson. (1990). *Shouting at the Wolf.* New York: Citadel Press.

Ring, Ken. (1980). *Life at Death.* New York: Coward, McCann & Geogehagan.

———. (1984). *Heading toward Omega.* New York: William Morrow.

———. (1992). *The Omega Project.* New York: William Morrow.

Ritchie, George. (1978). *Return from Tomorrow.* Waco, Tex.: Chosen.

Rivail, Hippolyte Léon Denizard. (1976) *The Spirits' Book.* (Anna Blackwell, Trans.) New York: Arno. (original work published 1875)

———. (1976) *The Mediums' Book.* (Anna Blackwell, Trans.) London: Psychic Press Ltd. (original work published 1876)

Rochas, Albert de. (1911). *Les Vies Successives.* Paris: Charcornal.

Rodewyk, Adolph. (1975). *Possessed by Satan.* (M. Ebon, Trans.). Garden City, N.Y.: Doubleday & Company. (original work published 1963)

Rogo, D. Scott. (1985). *The Search for Yesterday.* Englewood Cliffs, N.J.: Prentice-Hall.

———. (1987). *The Infinite Boundary.* New York: Dodd, Mead.

Ross, Colin. (1989). *Multiple Personality: Diagnosis, Clinical Features and Treatment.* New York: Wiley.

————. (1994). *The Osiris Complex.* Toronto: University of Toronto.

Russell, Jeffrey Burton. (1977). *The Devil: Perceptions of Evil from Antiquity to Primitive Christianity.* New York: Cornell University Press.

Sabom, Michael. (1982). *Recollections of Death.* New York: Harper & Row.

Sagan, Samuel. (1994). *Entities: Parasites of the Body of Energy.* Sydney, Australia: Clairvision School.

————. (1996). *Regression: Past-Life Therapy for Here and Now Freedom.* Sydney, Australia: Clairvision School.

Sargant, William. (1973). *The Mind Possessed.* New York: Penguin.

Schacter, Daniel. (2001). *The Seven Sins of Memory.* New York: Houghton Mifflin.

Schnabel, Jim. (1997). *Remote Viewers: The Secret History of America's Psychic Spies.* New York: Dell.

Schreiber, Flora Rheta. (1973). *Sybil.* Chicago: Regnery.

Schultz, Duane. (1981). *A History of Modern Psychology,* Third Edition. New York: Academic Press.

Singer, June. (1973). *Boundaries of the Soul: The Practice of Jung's Psychology.* New York: Doubleday.

Snow, Chet. (1989). *Mass Dreams of the Future.* New York: Doubleday.

Starr, Aloa. (1987). *Prisoners of Earth.* Los Angeles: Aura.

Steiner, Rudolf. (1968). *Life between Death and Rebirth.* New York: Anthroposophic Press.

Stevenson, Ian. (1974a). *Xenoglossy: A Review and Report of a Case.* Charlottesville: University Press of Virginia.

————. (1974b). *Twenty Cases Suggestive of Reincarnation.* Charlottesville: University Press of Virginia

————. (1984). *Unlearned Language: New Studies in Xenoglossy.* Charlottesville: University Press of Virginia.

————. (1997). *Where Reincarnation and Biology Intersect.* Westport, Conn.: Praeger.

Stone, Hal, and Sidra Winkelman. (1985). *Embracing Ourselves.* Marina del Rey, Calif.: DeVorss.

————. (1989). *Embracing Each Other.* San Rafael, Calif.: New World Library.

Strachey, J. (Ed.). (1953). *The Standard Edition of the Complete Psychological Works of Sigmund Freud* (Vol. 7). London: Hogarth Press.

Sutphen, Dick. (1976). *You Were Born Again to Be Together.* New York: Simon & Schuster.

———. (1978). *Past Lives, Future Loves.* New York: Simon & Schuster.

———. (1988). *Pre-Destined Love.* New York: Pocket Books.

———. (1982). *Unseen Influences.* New York: Pocket Books.

Swedenborg, Emanuel. (1979). *Heaven and Hell.* (G. F. Dole, Trans.). New York: Swedenborg Foundation. (original work published 1758)

Sylvia, Clare with William Novak. (1997). *Change of Heart.* New York: Little, Brown.

Taylor, Eugene. (1984). *William James on Exceptional Mental States: The 1896 Lowell lectures.* Amherst: University of Massachusetts.

TenDam, Hans. (1987). *Exploring Reincarnation.* (A. E. J. Wils, Trans.). New York: Penguin.

Thigpen, C., and H. Cleckly. (1957). *The Three Faces of Eve.* New York: Fawcett.

Van Dusen, Wilson. (1974). *The Presence of Other Worlds.* New York: Swedenborg Foundation.

Verney, Thomas. (1982). *The Secret Life of the Unborn Child.* New York: Dell.

———. (1987). *Pre- and Perinatal Psychology: An Introduction.* New York: Human Sciences.

Villoldo, Albert, and Stanley Krippner. (1986). *Healing States.* New York: Simon & Schuster.

Walsh, Roger, and Frances Vaughn, Eds. (1980). *Beyond Ego: Transpersonal Dimensions In Psychology.* Los Angeles: Tarcher.

Wambach, Helen. (1978). *Reliving Past Lives.* New York: Harper & Row.

———. (1979). *Life Before Life.* New York: Wm. Morrow.

Weiss, Brian. (1988). *Many Lives, Many Masters.* New York: Simon & Schuster.

White, John (Ed.). (1974). *Frontiers of Consciousness.* New York: Julian Press.

Whitfield, Charles. (1987). *Healing the Child Within.* Deerfield Beach, Fla.: Health Communications.

Whitton, Joel, and Joe Fisher. (1986). *Life Between Life.* New York: Doubleday.

Wickland, Carl. (1924). *Thirty Years Among the Dead.* Los Angeles: National Psychological Institute.

———. (1934). *The Gateway of Understanding.* Los Angeles: National Psychological Institute.

Woodward, M. (1985). *Scars of the Soul: Holistic Healing in the Edgar Cayce Readings.* Columbus, Ohio: Brindabella.

Woolger, Roger. (1987). *Other Lives, Other Selves.* New York: Doubleday.

Young, W. C. (1987). "Emergence of a Multiple Personality in a Post Traumatic Stress Disorder of Adulthood." *American Journal of Clinical Hypnosis,* 29, pp. 249–254.

Zuendel, Friedrich. (1999). *The Awakening: One Man's Battle with Darkness.* Farmington, Penn.: The Plough Publishing House.

Endnotes

Introduction

1. Charles Tart edited and produced the classic book on the subject of human consciousness. Sections of the book describe the effects of hypnosis, drugs, meditation, biofeedback, and dreams.

2. Albert de Rochas, *Les Vies Successive.* Col. de Rochas was one of the most eminent French psychic investigators before his death in 1914. While under hypnosis, several of his hypnotic subjects remembered past lives and furnished information about some distant town or location that was confirmed, while their claimed past-life identities could not be validated. In an article published in 1905, he mentioned that work similar to his had been conducted in Spain, but he cited no reference.

3. Asa Martin, *Researches in Reincarnation and Beyond.*

4. Dianetics, developed by Ron Hubbard, expanded into Scientology, a highly controversial organization that claimed to have methodologies useful in clearing mental, emotional, and physical problems. Past-life memories often emerge during the auditing procedures.

5. *You Have Been Here Before,* by Edith Fiore, Ph.D., 1978; *Past Lives Therapy,* by Morris Netherton, Ph.D, 1978; *You Were Born Again to Be Together,* 1976, and *Past Lives, Future Loves,* 1978, by Dick Sutphen; *Reliving Past Lives,* 1978, and *Life Before Life,* 1979, by Helen Wambach, Ph.D.

6. George Gallup, *Adventures in Immortality.*

7. American Psychiatric Association, *DSM-IV.*

8. Jon Klimo, *Channeling;* Arthur Hastings, *With the Tongues of Men and Angels.*

9. Nandor Fodor, *Encyclopedia of Psychic Science*, pp. 265–266.

10. Author Eugene Taylor, *William James on Exceptional Mental States: The 1896 Lowell Lectures*, has done much to stimulate interest in James's concept of "radical empiricism."

11. Frederic W. H. Myers wrote a major treatise on the subject, published posthumously in 1904, 1,360 pages in two volumes entitled *Human Personality and Its Survival of Bodily Death*. Myers died in 1901. These volumes still stand as the definitive work on the subject.

12. Clairvoyance (French, "clear seeing"), the ability to see into the ethereal realm without using physical eyes; psychic perception of visual images of people, places, and objects, and correct interpretation of the images. Clairaudience (French, "clear audio, or hearing"), the ability to receive sounds, words, sentences, and voices, with no apparent source. Clairsentience (French, "clear sensation or feeling"), the ability to perceive information by a "feeling within the whole body" without outer stimuli related to the sensation. These spiritual gifts of discernment, or psychic abilities, must be controlled by the individual in order to maintain firm grounding in mundane reality.

13. Stan Grof, M.D. has explored human consciousness perhaps more extensively than any other investigator. His books describe his work and many of these phenomena. See *Realms of the Human Unconscious* and *Beyond The Brain*.

14. See Olga Hoyt, *Exorcism*. The notion of possession, or control of a living being by a nonphysical consciousness, or entity, has been known or theorized in every time and every culture. The first recorded instance was found scratched on a clay tablet in Assyrian cuneiform text some 2,500 years ago.

Chapter 1

1. *The Demonologist*, by Gerald Brittle, 1980, described the work of Ed and Lorraine Warren, a Catholic couple who dealt with Earthbound souls and dark force entities as well. *Hostage to the Devil*, by Jesuit Malachi Martin, 1976, described five severe cases of demonic possession, written in a sensational, fear-provoking style that nearly caused me to abandon the work entirely. One of the first books I read on the subject, *Thirty Years Among the Dead*, by Dr. Carl Wickland, 1924, described only cases of possession by Earthbound spirits, and was the basis for the development of Spirit Releasement Therapy. Treatment of the DFEs developed a few years after I began investigating the phenomenon of spirit possession. Discovery of ETs and development of treatment followed that by a few more years.

2. Carl Wickland, *Thirty Years Among the Dead*, (1924), *Gateway to Understanding*, (1934).

3. William Finch, *The Pendulum and Possession*; Aloa Starr, *Prisoners of Earth*; Eugene Maurey, *Exorcism*.

4. E. Foulks, IONS Bulletin.

5. Hyslop, 1917; Wickland, 1924, 1934; Stevenson, 1974a, 1984; Allison, 1980; Guirdham, 1982; McAll, 1982; Crabtree, 1985; Fiore, 1987a,b; Villoldo and Krippner, 1986: Baldwin, 1992.

6. See appendix A.

7. William P. Blatty, *The Exorcist*; Tom Allen, *Possessed: The True Story of an Exorcism*.

8. Fiore, Guirdham, Maurey, Baldwin.

9. See Rosalyn Bruyere's fine work on the chakras, *Wheels of Light*.

10. Claire Sylvia (with William Novak), *A Change of Heart*, 1997, describes her experience of heart and lung transplant, following which she had a strong desire for chicken nuggets and beer. She questioned a number of people who might be considered as experts in consciousness, receiving numerous explanations for the phenomenon. She mentioned possession as a notion so preposterous that she could not even think about it. Within our model, it is the obvious cause of her behavior, and other people have discovered similar situations.

11. Adam Crabtree, *Multiple Man*.

12. See appendix C for the text of the Sealing Light Meditation.

13. J. MacDonald, *American Journal of Psychiatry*.

14. D. Barlow, G. Abel, and E. Blanchard reported this remarkable case in *Archives of Sexual Behavior*.

15. See Helen Wambach's fine book on the Planning Stage, *Life Before Life*.

16. See Dick Sutphen's *Unseen Influences*. In the front pages of his book Sutphen states, "It is time to reject the unseen influences and direct your own destiny." Good advice, good book.

17. Ralph Allison, *Minds in Many Pieces*; Adam Crabtree, *Multiple Man*; William J. Baldwin, *Spirit Releasement Therapy: A Technique Manual*.

18. See D. Scott Rogo, *The Infinite Boundary*. Rogo was a thorough investigator in the arena of the paranormal. This book presents a level-headed assessment of the condition termed "spirit possession."

19. This phenomenon is called apportation psychokinesis and involves dematerializing of an object or objects in one location and rematerializing them in another location, usually in the presence of the psychic or medium responsible for the event. Manning apparently was not doing this consciously. See June Bletzer's impressive and extensive volume, *The Donning International Encyclopedic Psychic Dictionary*, p. 32.

20. Matthew Manning, *The Link*.

21. Albert Villoldo and Stanley Krippner, *Healing States*.

22. Adam Crabtree's classic work, *Multiple Man*.

23. Jon Klimo, *Channelling*; Arthur Hastings, *With the Tongues of Men and Angels*.

24. The shadow is described as the darker personal side of each human being, that which is dreadful or evil and disapproved of by the conscious mind. This was theorized and described by the great psychiatrist, Carl Jung.

Chapter 2

1. Many books have been written in recent years on the inner child. Abrams, Bradshaw, Whitfield, and others have contributed to this field.

2. See appendix C.

3. Dr. Edith Fiore also discovered this same prevalence.

4. *Diagnosis and Treatment of the Spirit Possession Syndrome* was the first doctoral dissertation on the clinical treatment of this condition.

5. See the author's book, *Spirit Releasement Therapy: A Technique Manual,* Second Edition.

Chapter 3

1. *Roe v. Wade* was a landmark Supreme Court decision that allowed a woman the right to privacy in opting for abortion during the first six months of pregnancy. It has caused a great deal of emotional upset through the years and is still challenged by many pro-life groups. A life is destroyed by abortion. Is it medicine, or is it murder? A soul-wrenching question.

Chapter 4

1. See Eugene Taylor, *William James on Exceptional Mental States: The 1896 Lowell Lectures.*

2. See the section on Recovery of Soul-Mind Fragmentation in the author's SRT manual.

3. Robert Assagioli, *Psychosynthesis.*

4. Hal Stone and Sidra Winkelman, *Embracing Ourselves* and *Embracing Each Other.*

5. Abrams, Bradshaw, Whitfield.

6. Martha Crampton, "Psychosynthesis" in Corsini, *Handbook of Innovative Psychotherapies.*

7. F. Putnam, IONS Bulletin.

8. Robert J. Campbell's *Psychiatric Dictionary,* Fifth Edition, p. 458.

9. American Psychiatric Association, *Diagnostic and Statistical Manual of Mental Disorders,* Fourth Edition, p. 269–270.

10. Richard. P. Kluft, in B. G. Braun (Ed.), *Treatment of Multiple Personality Disorder.*

11. Sandra Ingerman, *Soul Retrieval.*

12. The Bible describes the silver cord that attaches the soul to the body (Ecclesiastes 12:6). A part of this cord, a silver thread, seems to remain connected with the separated fragment in most cases (Baldwin, 1992, p. 173).

13. Allison, 1980; McAll, 1982; Crabtree, 1985; Baldwin, 1992.

Chapter 5

1. C. S. Lewis, preface to *The Screwtape Letters.*

2. Jeffrey Burton Russell, *The Devil: Perceptions of Evil from Antiquity to Primitive Christianity.*

3. Shakuntala Modi, *Remarkable Healings.*

4. Friedrich Zuendel wrote a biography, published in 1999, describing the experience of a German minister, Johann Christoph Blumhardt (1805–1880). Blumhardt's own detailed report, entitled *An Account of Gottliebin Dittus' Illness,* tells the story of an exorcism that became an ordeal lasting more than a year, but with very successful deliverance and healing of the young woman. For me, a most intriguing point in Zuendel's book was: "In general, most of the demons that showed themselves in Möttlingen

between August 1842 and December 1843 desperately yearned for liberation from the bonds of Satan" (p. 49).

5. John Warwick Montgomery, *Demon Possession*; Jeffrey Burton Russell, *The Devil: Perceptions of Evil from Antiquity to Primitive Christianity*; Matthew Linn and Dennis Linn, *Deliverance Prayer*.

6. Kelly, *The Devil, Demonology and Witchcraft*.

7. Father Francis MacNutt describes this notion in his book *Healing*, p. 196.

8. *Encarta 98 Desk Encyclopedia* and *1996–97* Microsoft Corporation. All rights reserved.

9. Ignorance comes from the root word "ignore," and has nothing to do with stupidity or lack of intelligence.

Chapter 6

1. This process is described in detail in the author's book, *Spirit Releasement Therapy: A Technique Manual*, pp. 323–349.

2. The Bible.

Chapter 7

1. In her book *Encounters*, psychologist Edith Fiore, Ph.D. describes a case of an attachment by an ET. Her client, a man in his mid-forties, was a little boy at the time of the attachment, walking along a dirt road in Washington state. The nonphysical alien swooped down toward Earth, discovered the boy, and simply came into the back of his head. The boy was unaware of the intrusion. It seems the alien came to Earth, as had many others of its kind, to find a retirement sanctuary. He randomly chose this boy as his resting place, his nest.

2. Dr. Roger Leir, *The Aliens and the Scalpel*.

3. This and other ET cases are described in detail in the author's book, *CE-VI: Close Encounters of the Possession Kind*.

Chapter 8

1. Infantile amnesia is described in Freud's collected works, edited by Strachey.

2. David Chamberlain, *Babies Remember Birth*; Thomas Verney, *The Secret Life of the Unborn Child*; Morris Netherton, *Past Lives Therapy*.

3. For an intense in-depth look at birth and its effect on our lives, Stan Grof's book, *Beyond the Brain*, is not to be missed.

4. Morris Netherton, *Past Lives Therapy*.

Chapter 9

1. Voltaire, quoted in *Old Truths in a New Light* by Lady Caithness (London, 1876).

2. J. Head and S. Cranston have produced an amazing body of work in their three books: *Reincarnation: An East-West Anthology; Reincarnation in World Thought;* and *Reincarnation: The Phoenix Fire Mystery*. Sylvia Cranston and Carey Williams continued with *Reincarnation: A New Horizon in Science, Religion, and Society*.

3. Ian Stevenson refers to these cases as "suggestive of reincarnation."

4. Ian Stevenson, *Where Reincarnation and Biology Intersect.*

5. June Bletzer has compiled an extensive volume of esoteric, psychic, and spiritual knowledge, *The Donning International Encyclopedic Psychic Dictionary.*

6. In his book, *Exploring Reincarnation,* Dutch past-life therapist Hans TenDam uses the term "life plan" instead of my term, "Lifescript." He suggests the term "life retrospect" for the Review Stage.

7. Helen Wambach, *Life Before Life.* Wambach regressed several thousand people in small and large groups. Her research revealed a broad consistency in the reports of such details reported by people across the country.

8. Joel Whitton and Joe Fisher, *Life Between Life.* Some of Whitton's clients described a judgment board of elevated spirit guides, from three to twelve in number, conducting the review and later assisting in developing the plan for the next life. Most souls require a detailed blueprint of the coming life, advanced souls need only an outline.

9. See Michael Newton, *Journey of Souls* and *Destiny of Souls,* for a detailed look at the space between lives. Newton writes of his client's descriptions of the Council of Elders, who review our life just passed and assist in the planning of the next incarnation.

10. Head and Cranston, 1977, *Reincarnation: The Phoenix Fire Mystery* pp. 156–160. Reincarnation was voted out of religious doctrine, therefore out of the spiritual reality. The only way to gain the grace of God was through the Church fathers, unlike the system of personal responsibility inherent in the philosophy of karma and reincarnation as expressed in Buddhism.

11. Quincy Howe Jr., *Reincarnation for the Christian.*

12. Transpersonal refers to experience in which an individual transcends the limitations of identifying exclusively with the body, ego, or personality, such as extrasensory perception, out-of-body experience, Jung's notion of collective consciousness. Also included are mythical, archetypal, and symbolic realms of inner experience that can come through dreams and imagery (Frances Vaughn in *Beyond Ego*). Jung held that all products of the unconscious are symbolic.

13. See *Lifetimes,* by Dr. Fredrick Lenz, which details the cases of 128 people who had waking experiences of past lives.

14. Carolyn Myss authored *Anatomy of the Spirit,* essential reading for healers of any and all orientations.

15. June Bletzer describes the astral body as invisible, ethereal substance interpenetrating the physical body and extending beyond the body five to eight inches. Following death, the astral body envelopes the soul consciousness in the etheric or nonphysical world. The etheric double also interpenetrates and surrounds the body with a higher frequency of vibration. Serves as a pattern for one's future lifestyle in this or a future incarnation. These spirit or energy bodies are visible to the newly deceased soul, as narrated by the client in altered state.

16. Karma and reincarnation cannot be separated. Karma is a concept that refers to the cosmic ledger, the balance sheet of personal deeds and debts to others. All debts will be balanced before we go home to God in the

final step of spiritual evolution. These karmic debts can be paid in suffering, balanced with good works, erased through wisdom, or canceled by Grace.

17. Future-life progressions are described in *Past Lives, Future Lives* by Bruce Goldberg, D.D.S., and *Mass Dreams of the Future*, by Chet Snow, Ph.D.

18. Helen Wambach, *Reliving Past Lives*.

19. Chet Snow, *Mass Dreams of the Future*.

20. Frederick Lenz, *Lifetimes*.

21. American Psychiatric Association *DSM-IV*, pp. 424–429; H. Hendin and A. P. Haas, *Wounds of War: The Psychological Aftermath of Combat in Vietnam*.

Chapter 10

1. Ruth Brandon's *The Spiritualists*.

2. Ibid.

3. Carl Wickland, *Thirty Years Among the Dead* and *The Gateway of Understanding*.

4. Titus Bull, *Analysis of Unusual Experience in Healing Relative to Diseased Minds*.

5. Eugene Taylor, *William James on Exceptional Mental States: The 1896 Lowell Lectures*.

6. Moody, Kübler-Ross, Ring, Atwater, Grey, Sabom, Morse, Rawlings, and Ritchie.

7. George Gallup, *Adventures in Immortality*.

8. George Ritchie, *Return from Tomorrow*.

Chapter 11

1. See *The Portable Jung*, edited by Joseph Campbell.

2. See books by Rabbi Yonassan Gershom, *Beyond the Ashes* and *From Ashes to Healing*; and Maryanne Clare, *The Splintered Soul*.

3. Steven Levenkron, *Treating and Overcoming Anorexia Nervosa*.

4. Morris Netherton, *Past Lives Therapy*.

5. Trevor Ravenscroft has researched and chronicled this period in history in his books, *The Spear of Destiny* and *The Mark of The Beast*, with Tim Wallace-Murphy.

Chapter 13

1. Jon Klimo, *Channeling*.

2. Schwarz, Harary, Puthoff, and Targ established the field of remote viewing at SRI, Stanford Research Institute. Jim Schnabel's book, *Remote Viewers: The Secret History of America's Psychic Spies* is a very clear exposition of remote viewing. Joe McMoneagle's book, *Mind Trek*, is an excellent personal account by one of the best remote viewers produced by the U.S. Army.

3. Larry Dossey, author of *Healing Words: The Power of Prayer and the Practice of Medicine*, gathered information on the power of prayer in remote healing. He was surprised to find well-documented studies showing the undeniable results of prayer, even when the receivers were unaware of the prayer being directed to them.

4. See *Quantum Reality* by Nick Herbert.

5. Universal oneness or universal consciousness is considered to be the divine consciousness, the one total awareness that is conscious of being. Everything in the universe (or universes) is a part of, and belongs to, the "one" consciousness of being. Every animate and inanimate thing consists of consciousness, some of lesser, some of greater degree; the universal awareness is distributed in all things, unevenly, in accordance with the nature of the thing, each with enough awareness to know its "function." Everything is aware that it is connected to the mother consciousness, and to some this awareness of connection is more acute. From Bletzer's *Encyclopedic Psychic Dictionary* (p. 658).

6. See chapter 24 of Ross's book, *The Osiris Complex.*

Chapter 14

1. William James, *Principles of Psychology, Vol. 1*, 1950, pp. 391–393.

2. Walter Young in *American Journal of Clinical Hypnosis*, 29, 249–254.

Epilogue

1. The International Association for Regression Research and Therapies (IAART) can be reached at P.O. Box 20151, Riverside, CA 20151. The inspiration for the organization and founding president was Hazel Denning, Ph.D., to whom this book is dedicated, with deep and abiding love, respect, and gratitude.

2. George Gallup, *Adventures in Immortality.*

3. These thoughts were expressed in his 1690 work, *Essay Concerning Human Understanding.* Locke founded the school of empiricism, which emphasizes the importance of the senses in pursuit of knowledge rather than intuition or logical deduction. Opposed to empiricism is rationalism, which asserts that the mind is capable of recognizing reality by means of reason, a faculty that exists independent of experience.

4. As a young man, Dr. Stevenson knew that his personal convictions about reincarnation would be scoffed at by professionals. He chose medical school, the specialty of psychiatry, and a university post as a platform from which to bring his ideas to the world. His research into the possibilities is thorough and methodical, and is considered sound by his peers. (Personal communication)

5. Stevenson's book, *Where Reincarnation and Biology Intersect*, contains fascinating cases gathered over thirty years of investigation. Earlier works also described the birthmark phenomena.

6. See the many books by Dick Sutphen.

7. Wilder Penfield's final book, *The Mystery of the Mind*, was a brilliant synopsis of his life's work, written in simple style with beautiful clarity for every reader. He revealed himself as a spiritual man who had searched for some scientific evidence of mind, something greater in mankind. Clearly, he believed in mind-to-mind communication, in particular the mind of man and the mind of God.

8. Stan Grof also describes this phenomenon in his book, *Beyond the Brain.*

9. Dr. Samuel Sagan, Australian psychiatrist and founder of the Clairvision School, suggests the astral body, which carries the scars of the soul (also known as *samskaras*), is the human soul. See *Regression: Past-Life Therapy for Here and Now Freedom.*

10. M. Woodward, *Scars of the Soul.*

11. See Daniel Schacter's book, *The Seven Sins of Memory.*

12. Candace Pert's book, *Molecules of Emotion,* makes fascinating reading. Her discoveries shook some foundation blocks of medicine and psychology, and were largely ignored by the health professions. So much more could be accomplished by the clinical application of her findings.

13. Hall and Nordby, *A Primer of Jungian Psychology.*

14. David Deutsch, Ph.D., winner of the Paul Dirac Medal and Prize, author of *The Fabric of Reality,* is a leading theoretical physicist who is the most eloquent spokesman of the Many Universes interpretation of quantum behavior. He argues that we are much closer to a Theory of Everything than we realize.

15. See the article, "Quantum Shmantum," by Tim Folger in *Discover* magazine, September 2001.

16. Nick Herbert, *Quantum Reality;* Brian Greene, *The Elegant Universe.*

17. Coleman, Butcher, and Carlson, 1980, pp. 25–44.

18. Clark Moustakas' *Heuristic Research.* From the introduction:

> The root meaning of *heuristic* comes from the Greek *heuriskein* meaning to discover or to find. It refers to a process of internal search through which one discovers the nature and meaning of experience and develops methods and procedures for further investigation and analysis. The self of the researcher is present throughout the process and, while understanding the phenomenon with increasing depth, the researcher also experiences growing self-awareness and self-knowledge. Heuristic processes incorporate creative self-processes and self-discoveries.
>
> The cousin word of heuristics is *eureka,* exemplified by the Greek mathematician Archimedes' discovery of a principle of buoyancy. . . . The process of discovery leads investigators to new images and meanings regarding human phenomena, but also to realizations relevant to their own experiences and lives.

Appendix B

1. *The American Heritage College Dictionary.* Boston: Houghton Mifflin. 1993, p. 797–798.

2. Ibid., p. 395.

Index

Index

About the Author

William J. Baldwin, Ph.D., is the author of four previous books including *Spirit Releasement Therapy* (Headline Books, 1992), *CE-VI: Close Encounters of the Possession Kind* (Headline Books, 1999), and *Past Life Therapy* (Headline Books, 2002). He is co-director of the Center for Human Relations in Enterprise, Florida, just outside of Orlando.

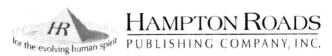

HAMPTON ROADS
PUBLISHING COMPANY, INC.

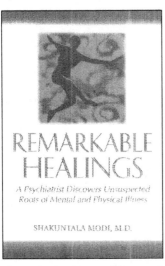

Remarkable Healings

A Psychiatrist Discovers Unsuspected Roots of Mental and Physical Illness

Shakuntala Modi, M.D.

While most doctors agree that emotional states affect our health, few would give credence to spiritual influences. However, Dr. Modi shows that many patients, under hypnosis, claimed to have spirits attached to their bodies and energy fields, creating psychological and physical problems. Dr. Modi describes techniques that release these spirits, revealing how patients can sometimes recover within a few sessions.

Paperback • 632 pages • ISBN 1-57174-079-1 • $19.95

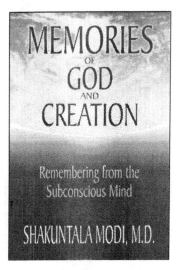

Memories of God and Creation
Remembering from the Subconscious Mind
Shakuntala Modi, M.D.

According to Dr. Modi, everyone carries memories of God and creation in their subconscious. This book presents information from many of her hypnotized patients including real descriptions of what it's like to be one with God, where evil comes from, how angels were created, how dying feels, and more.

Paperback • 304 pages • ISBN 1-57174-196-8 • $16.95

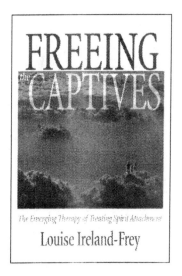

Freeing the Captives
The Emerging Therapy of Treating Spirit Attachment
Louise Ireland-Frey, M.D.

Dr. Ireland-Frey draws from her most interesting and dynamic cases in her more than two decades as a hypnotherapist to reveal how "attached" entities can be responsible for any number of physical, mental, and emotional disorders; what conditions make such invasions possible; what's meant by the terms obsession and possession—and what can be done to prevent them; and how to rescue lost and wandering souls.

Paperback • 346 pages • ISBN 1-57174-136-4 • $13.95